GENERAL PRINCIPLES AND PRACTICE OF PHLEBOTOMY

By Nicky J Pearce
MD (AM), ND, MH, BSc, ITEC, IHBC,
IIHHT, VTCT, ILM, AET, FBIAHA, FRCND,.
NATUROPATHIC DOCTOR & AESTHETICS TEACHER

This book is dedicated to my son Jake George.

This book is designed and written to accompany an accredited certificate course run at www.uchsc.co.uk

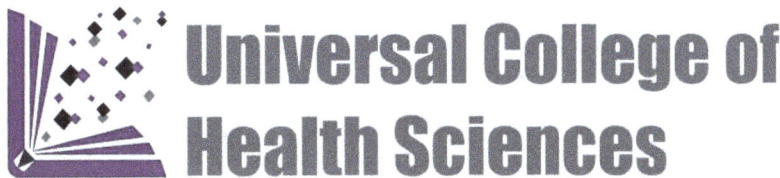

DISCLAIMER AND COPY RIGHTS

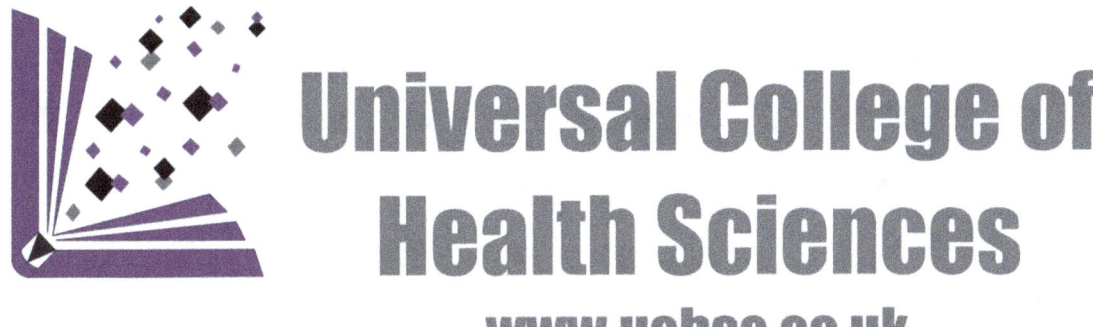

Contents

BY NICKY PEARCE

INTRODUCTION;

You may be wanting to undertake the study of phlebotomy for a number of reasons. You may be studying a health care qualification such as nursing, medicine, podiatry, physiotherapy, etc, and wish to lay the foundations in this area.

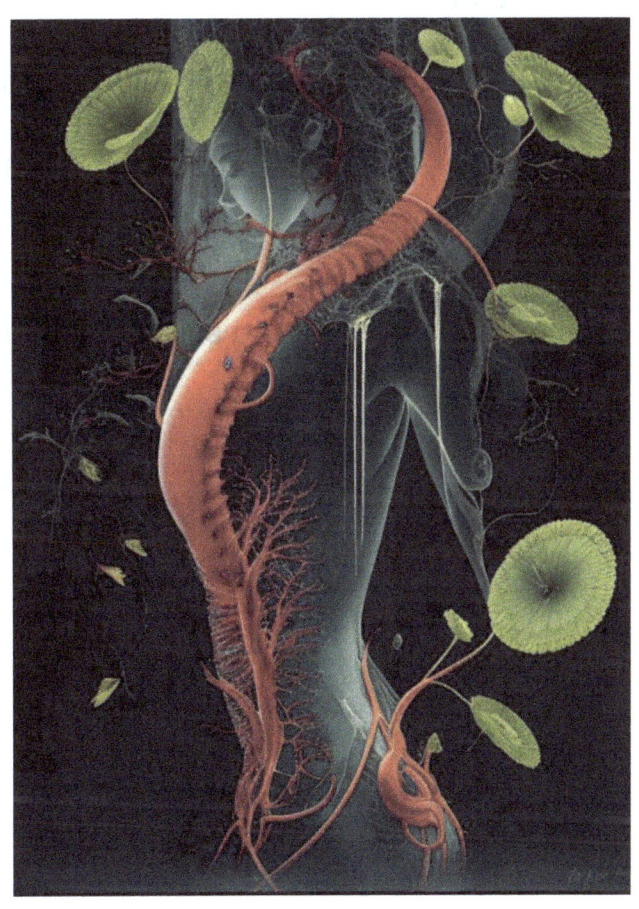

You may want to explore the possibilities or wish to take this up as a career either in the NHS, private clinics or even as a private phlebotomist working in your own clinic, subcontracted and or visiting people's homes taking blood for private testing services etc.

Whatever the reason, this book will equip you with some of the basics you will need to know to become safe, competent, reflective, accountable and independent professional phlebotomist practitioners.

For ease and fullness of explanations within this book, I will assume that you are either wanting to undertake phlebotomy for medical reasons, in which case there aren't technically any contra-indications to having the procedure done.

You will need to be careful with certain patients and take special precautions, for example, patients who are on anticoagulant drugs (blood thinners).

These patients tend to bleed for longer and bruise easily. So any patient who is on Warfarin, Heparin, and even Aspirin should be aware that their clotting times will be increased and they will need to hold the cotton wool to the puncture site after phlebotomy for a lot longer than usual.

If the patient can do so, they can do this whilst you attend to your administration. If not, and they are ill, as patients usually are when in hospitals, then you will have to be patient and do it for them.

If in any doubt you should always check with your supervisor, nurse or doctor.

Remember that blood tests are used to help diagnose medical conditions and are therefore essential for the patient to get done in a timely manner so that they can get treated and get better as soon as possible, cutting down the stress of the situation.

BY NICKY PEARCE

AIMS OF THIS BOOK;

To lay the foundations of relevant underpinning theory, and understanding so that the candidate can then go on to undertake practical training, initially on simulation arms, and then onto real live patients.

So as to develop the clinical skills required of a safe, competent, reflective, accountable and independent phlebotomy practitioner who is a valuable part of a team of healthcare professionals, and who can practice autonomously and safely.

Please also see the course descriptor that is issued and updated accordingly by UCHSc or any other institution you are studying at.

Always keep up to date and adhere to any relevant laws, policies and procedures where ever you are from. For example, policies, and procedures may vary in the UK from NHS trust to NHS trust. One trust may allow you to perform additional services such as cannulation, whereas the other may not. It is up to you as a professional and ethical practitioner to stay within the policies, procedures and any laws where you live and practice professionally.

This book that accompanies the UCHSc course is mapped to level 3 (A, Level), standards in the UK and for approximately 50 credits minimum of CPD points which is equivalent to 50 hours of theoretical study.

Extra credits can be awarded for practical training and further clinical supervision and assessment of successful blood draws.

HISTORY OF PHLEBOTOMY;

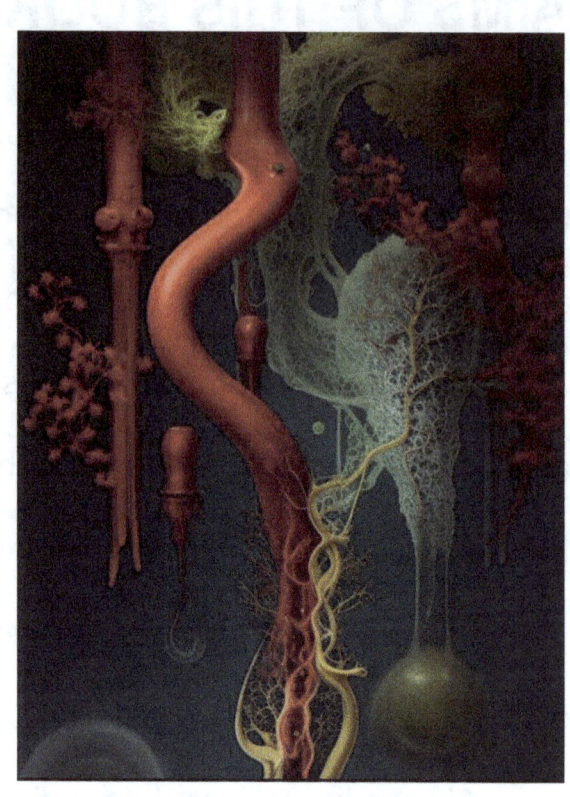

Phlebotomy from the Greek words Phlebos = vein and Temnein = to cut) has been around for over five millenniums. Is the act of drawing blood from the circulatory system by either a small cut or puncture.

In the past, it was done by incision/cut and was called bloodletting. It is thought that it was first practised in Egypt around 1000 BC.

They thought by ridding the body of toxic blood would help release diseases, and evidence of this can be found in the Ebers Papyrus, where bloodletting and scarification was an accepted procedure.

In Greece, a prominent physician called Galen Pergamon, discovered that arteries as well as veins had blood. It was previously thought that the arteries were filled with air.

At this time they didn't know that blood circulated around the body, and instead, they thought that it just stagnated in our extremities.

During this period in history, many physicians also prescribed emetics to encourage vomiting and purging. Galen developed a complex system which would determine the location and quantity of blood to be let according to the disease.

He thought that blood should be let as close to the area of concern so that diseased/toxic blood could be purged from the body, and the disease with it.

The pilgrims were credited with taking Phlebotomy to the USA from Europe in the 18th century. It was common practice in these times to insert lancets into multiple locations along veins, withdrawing up to 4 pints of blood.

Over time other equipment was developed to improve the technique and its safety.

Bloodletting was popular for over a hundred years until it fell out of fashion in light of many harmful and deadly incidents over the years.

Bloodletting was a standard treatment for fevers in the 18th century. It was also popular for hypertension, comas, and drowsy headaches.

Bleeding was recommended for inflammation of the lungs, bounding pulses and difficulty in breathing. It was common practice to remove as much as 210 ounces were bled over a period of 6 days.

On December 13th 1799 George Washington took ill with a severe throat infection, it is alleged that three physicians were called in, and a total of 2365 ml or 2.36 litres of blood was drawn over a 12-hour period. George Washington eventually succumbed and died on the 14th. Nobody is sure whether it was from the infection or the massive amount of blood lost.

During the American civil war between 1861 and 1865, military physicians, unable to cope with the widespread infections, bled Union soldiers and civilians alike.

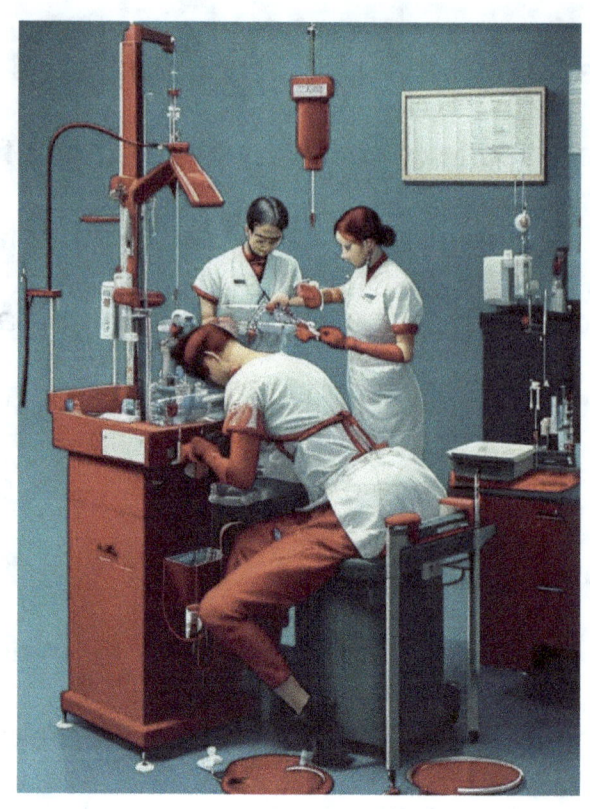

Early instruments included virtually anything sharp like stones, quills or animal teeth. The thumb lancet was introduced in the fifteenth century. It was a double-edged instrument, often with ornate handles made out of turtle shells.

Eventually, Lois Pasteur and Robert Koch conclusively proved that inflammations resulted from infection and thus, proved bloodletting was of no use in treating infections.

They offered a scientific explanation e.g. bacteria and researched possible treatments.

In 2008 three Kashmiri hospitals were reported to be using leeches, primarily to bleed patients as treatment for cardiac problems, arthritis, gout, chronic headaches and sinusitis.

Specially bred sterile leeches are used in modern medicine to drain hepatomas and reduce inflammation and oedema.

BY NICKY PEARCE

Historical records (Hired medicinal) indicate that leeches were used in medical treatment and date back to ancient Egypt and Greece. Bloodletting became popular in Victorian times in Britain, and used over 42 million leeches a year, creating an industry worth over £1 million. At 19th century prices.

Bloodletting was eventually called into question during the 18th century after a cascade of incidents, and it eventually fell out of favour.

Although extreme bloodletting was eventually seen as harmful, is it still practised today for a range of certain medical conditions e.g. Hemochromatosis. It is also still practised in cupping therapy particularly Hijama by Muslim people.

This is undertaken today using sterile pre-packed, single-use medical equipment e.g. needles and syringes. This equipment is also used to introduce or give intravenously medications and fluids for therapeutic purposes.

Phlebotomy nowadays is used to withdraw blood samples which are processed and tested in a medical laboratory to monitor and diagnose diseases.

It is also used in blood transfusion services. Although medical professionals are trained to undertake this service, most don't have the time. So they have chosen to designate this to trained professional phlebotomists who specialise in this procedure.

Phlebotomists work in a wide range of settings, from clinics, health centres, hospitals, labs, scientific research, home visits, and even in private practice contracted by other health care professionals.

Phlebotomy is a truly flexible and rewarding career choice for some. You can work in the NHS or private health care facilities, or with other medical professionals or aesthetic practitioners doing Platelet Rich Plasma and Vampire facials for example.

You could work with Biobanks, who attend births to take samples from placentas to store in Biobanks for potential later use if the child becomes ill, or for other purposes in the future such as growing organs and treating cancers.

Phlebotomists could work with natural health practitioners taking their client's blood and sending them off for testing at private laboratories, or even work with laboratories directly.

Further training and education in health and care or even going to college or university to study as a health professional.

You are only limited by your imagination as to how you design your career so that you experience the best work, life and career aspirations to the full.

BY NICKY PEARCE

WORKFLOW CYCLES AND MINIMISING ERRORS;

Workflow cycles are important within the phlebotomy profession, because getting blood samples back to the lab for testing may be time-dependent.

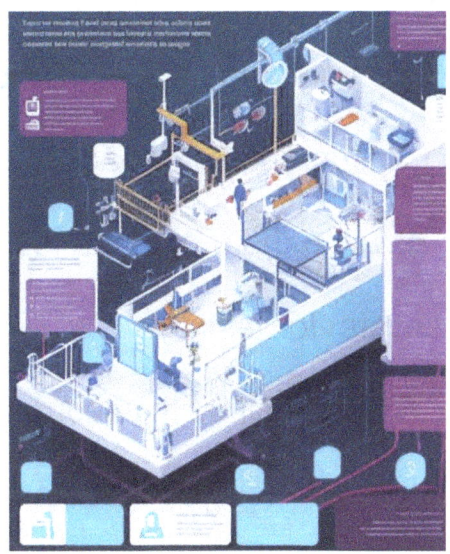

The fresher the sample the better, and more accurate for testing purposes.

Therefore having a positive effect on patient diagnosis, treatment and overall care.

Also for the accuracy of some tests as well. Certain samples may need to be returned to the lab within a certain time limit, and if they're not then you risk having to undertake the procedure again. Putting the patient through more pain, anxiety and stress, making them have the procedure done again, and having to wait for diagnosis and appropriate treatments, which could potentially be dangerous!

When you turn up for your shift you should plan your day according to the draws you are to perform and in order of urgency.

You triage patients, or this may be done for you according to the urgency of the test. So that you undertake the procedures from patients in an orderly fashion according to freshness requirements, especially if you are the one that is responsible for transporting the samples back to the lab.

You must make sure that everything is clearly labelled using a perm marker, and in accordance with the requirements, and then booked into the system immediately upon returning back to the lab.

Your job may therefore also entail not just undertaking the procedures, but also transporting them back to the lab, putting them into the computer system, and then passing them onto the technicians or medical laboratory scientific officers (Scientists) for testing.

This will all be in accordance with your job description, induction and training you receive when you first start and as you progress in your career. As you progress in your career you may also be trained to undertake additional procedures such as cannulation, paediatric blood draws etc.

A phlebotomist will be seeing patients of all ages and in all states of health.

You must be mindful of your actions and words at this sensitive time to your patients and others around you.

Be professional, and be straight to the point. Be reassuring, yet detach yourself so as not to get transference from patients.

Remember it is your job to take blood, and that is it. Unless you are a qualified healthcare professional involved in the patient's diagnosis, and treatment you should refrain from commenting on such things as test results or medical conditions.

BY NICKY PEARCE

As a phlebotomist you will see very anxious patients who may be frightened of getting blood taken or frightened of needles, and also the results that they may provide. This is where your empathy, reassurance and seamless phlebotomy skills are coveted.

If you need any help whilst undertaking the procedures you should ask another staff member e.g. your supervisor, or nurse etc.

You should aim to get in and out smoothly, and timely so as not to cause any more anxiety or stress to the patient, and also to help with your workflow. Some patients can be talkative and lonely, be nice yet undertake the procedure within an appropriate time, or you will be thrown off your schedule and this may affect results and cause more errors as previously mentioned.

Each time you go to work, you will pick up your list of patients, and the tests that they require.

You can set up your trolley or case appropriately with equipment, supplies, sharps containers and administration (paperwork). Decide which order to see the patients (Triage if this isn't already done for you), and then off you go.

Always have extra equipment and supplies on hand, just in case you need them.

Before using any cleanser on your patient always check, and ask them if they are allergic to anything. Some patients may be allergic to latex gloves, so use nitrile instead. Some may be allergic to chlorhexidine so don't use anything with that in.

Just ask, or if you can't then check with the nurse or doctor beforehand. If in a hospital it may be posted behind the bed or in the patient notes at the foot of the bed, you can check the allergies section first.

Needle stick injury Stats and video here. If you have a needle stick injury you should follow the procedure in the following video and then report it to the appropriate person, complete any report forms and you may be referred to occupational health for testing, prophylactic vaccination and Post Exposure Prophylaxis using antivirals to prevent HIV infection.

If you are self-employed you should attend your GP or local A&E for this as soon as possible.

WHO guidelines on drawing blood. Best practices in phlebotomy. 109-page document that can be downloaded from the WHO website.

You should always download or obtain any other guidelines policies and procedures from your country, state, medical supervisor, or any other relevant authorities, and keep up to date with any developments and changes through continual professional development and reflective practice etc.

This will help increase your workflow cycle, accuracy, fewer mistakes, and safety for you and those on whom you perform phlebotomy.

BY NICKY PEARCE

PROFESSIONAL STUDIES

When undertaking the professional practice of Phlebotomy, there are many other concerns to be taken into account to be a safe, competent, accountable and reflective professional practitioner.

Consideration, learning and assimilation of these are the things that will set you apart as a professional.

I'm my opinion this topic deserves to be a full course in its own right, as it's subject areas are so vast and wide-ranging.

You need to learn a lot of things in order to become a professional in the health and or aesthetics field, but this kind of subjects that I will discuss here are usually left alone or just glossed over superficially, unless you are undertaking some regulated qualification accredited by the government.

By just glossing over this leaves the learner with gaps that can be really important to close, and they're left to their own devices to study the subjects that they think they need, which they may, or may not need.

So to prevent you from wasting time studying a lot of subjects that you probably won't need I have put together this very brief section on professional studies. I advise you to read around and do more research on this topic, especially regarding legal and licensure aspects in your location.

PROFESSIONAL ETHICS

As a professional you will need to be aware of some core subjects that are involved in guiding your professional practice. Ethically and legally you have a duty of care for those you work with, treat, your colleagues and your own health, safety and legal practice.

Ignorance is no self-defence in the eyes of the law! The best way to establish some basic foundations with regard to your professional practice is to join some kind of professional association. This may be voluntary or mandatory.

In the UK for example it is voluntary, and there are many different private non-governmental associations you can choose from. You just have to find the right one for your needs. In the USA, for example, in some states, you may need to become licensed and join a state-approved professional association.

These professional associations will issue their members with licenses, registrations, certificates and a handbook of professional ethics and standards to which they are bound legally. This means that the practitioner can be expected to practice to a set of specified standards to protect the profession, the association, the public and the individual practitioner.

You should always read the member's handbook so that you know these standards and policies and procedures for various things such as if you need insurance if you need to undertake continual professional development courses, discipline procedures, complaints etc.

Your professional association may offer lots of different services e.g.

Maintain a register and issue licenses. Offering accreditation to course providers, or holding national or internal or external exams.

Offer insurance of different kinds with discounts and legal advice.

Provide a code of professional ethics and safety standards.

Provide complaints and disciplinary procedures to hold members accountable.

Provide marketing, promotion and networking activities and events.

For example, this course is accredited by the British and International Association of Health and Aesthetics (B.I.A.H.A.). Upon graduation, you will be granted automatic registration and licensure for 1 year.

This is included as part of your learning contract with the college, you sign to say you agree to be bound by its policies, procedures, standards, ethics etc. But additionally, you are also bound by its accrediting organisation rules the B.I.A.H.A.

TASK:- Go and have a look around the internet and check out the rules for registration and licensure in your field and in your location. What is available? And download a copy of the handbook or rules if you can.

THE CONSULTATION PROCESS

For any professional, this is one of the most important parts of your interaction with your patient or client. It's where you build trust through professionalism. This process is also slightly different for each practitioner of each different type.

For example, a foot health professional will involve more medical, surgical, and pharmacological history, a biomechanics assessment and more, so you need to know a lot more to be able to undertake this. Whereas for a Phlebotomist, especially in a hospital you would be performing this no matter what usually, because it's required to make a diagnosis or monitor medical conditions or therapies.

This process is used for many different reasons but for all professionals will follow a similar progression for the same reasons.

As a general rule, the consultation starts with the client/patient filling in a form, or they may already have an existing record which you may need to refer to, to check it over. In a hospital, some things will be posted above a patient's bed for staff such as nurses, assistants, and phlebotomists to see immediately.

As a phlebotomist you will be performing a procedure on the request of someone else, but you still need to make the required safety checks, not just for the patients benefit, but for your own health and safety, as you may need additional PPE if they have infectious disease and may need special precautions or barrier nursing techniques etc.

You're still an autonomous practitioner and will be held accountable for your professional practice, so you still need to check everything is ok, and follow the proper policies and procedures in your location.

Consultation is used to gather information on clients/patients for administration, marketing, promotion, and gather stats for advertising etc, if you run your own private practice.

It is also used to identify clients/patients who may be contra-indicated to having the procedure done. As we have already discussed, in hospitals and medical environments, contra-indications will not be considered much, because it is essential that the receive the service as part of their diagnosis and treatment.

However when Phlebotomy is undertaken for voluntary reasons such as if you are in private practice, you will need to take these into account.

Some contra-indications could be; clients/patients on anticoagulant drugs. In a hospital you would still have to do the procedure, but in private practice you can assess whether the benefits outweigh the risks involved. Risk being bleeding control.

When your patient is in a hospital surrounded by lots of medical staff. In your private clinic, there may not be any available to help out, so you may decide it's a risk or contra-indication you don't want to take. Cuts, bruises, swelling, pain, infections, thrombophlebitis etc, in the area where you want to undertake the procedure.

This is your time to be supportive, as they may be going through a tough time. Try not, however, to let them distract you or waffle and distract you from your workflow cycle. This is a fine balance.

If you're in private practice it's important to develop a rapport so that you encourage them to come back or even recommend your services to their family or friends. Getting business by word of mouth is the best kind.

During the consultation, it is important to document everything and write everything down in accordance with the accepted standards, and laws e.g. data protection act, privacy and confidentiality.

Remember that these documents are legal documents which could be requested in a court of law, should the need arise. So be careful what you write!

There will be a range of administration you will need to undertake, including written forms, computer databases etc. Don't forget to get signature of clients/patients or witnesses where appropriate etc.

TASK:- Download a copy of a consultation form or a test request form, and have a look at its format and the information printed on them.

Maybe even make your own if you are thinking of going into private practice.

BY NICKY PEARCE

BODY DYSMORPHIC DISORDER (BDD)

As a phlebotomist in a hospital health care setting this situation won't be in your remit. However, if you are thinking of doing Phlebotomy in a cosmetic surgery, aesthetic or beauty clinic, you should be aware of this subject.

Beauty comes in many shapes, sizes, and colours and it should be celebrated as such. Unfortunately for some people, they never see their true beauty. They see other people, but never their own. It's like we're all great at giving advice to others, but we never listen to ourselves.

Body dysmorphic disorder (BDD) is a growing concern, thought to effect 2.4% of the population, and it really should be taken seriously because it can make people anxious, depressed, and suicidal in extreme cases. It has a complex and individual aetiology for everyone that has it. It can exhibit in lesser or great amounts in an individual depending.

In the last few decades we have seen it increasing because of celebrities and the growth of social media putting out false lifestyles and expectations, pressuring people to look a certain way, or have a certain treatment because some famous person had it done.

BDD can start from a very young age when children are exposed to peer pressure in fashions, and looks. Everyone wants the latest trainers, jeans, tops, jewellery, botox, fillers, cosmetic surgery etc. It can become obsessive and mostly baseless feelings of being fat, ugly, too tall, too short, different race, or body image which can be reinforced by peer pressure, and bullying at school, and even at home.

Siblings and parents unknowingly or well meaningly trying to reverse psychology which eventually backfires and causes the child more psychological damage, which then transfers into adulthood because they weren't resolved.

It is natural to want to be and look the best we can in order to attract our soulmate.

However, because of BDD, this can go too far. BDD may be obvious when the person will do things like lock themselves away, withdraw and become introverted. Some become obsessed with changing their appearance.

BDD can occur later in life when people get rejected in one way or another.

We live in a throw away society, everyone has an opinion, and sometimes these opinions hurt. The grass is always greener, so when you get rejected or bullied a number of times through no fault of your own, and usually someone else insecurities, these doubts build up. Especially when alleged faults are found with your appearance and personality, and its natural to want to change this, to be part of the group. The problem is that cosmetic and aesthetic procedures can be addictive.

There are a number of factors which increase the risk of developing BDD. A family history. Negative body image. Perfectionism. Negative life experiences such as bullying or teasing as previously mentioned. Introversion, and media influences.

Common symptoms include; Extreme preoccupation with a perceived flaw in your physical appearance that to everyone else is nothing to worry about. attempting to hide the perceived flaw with makeup, clothes and seeking cosmetic surgery. Avoiding social situations because you feel extremely self-conscious. Constantly comparing your apparent flaw with others. Always seeking assurance about your appearance from others, even in a sneaky way. Low self-esteem.

Compulsive behaviours such as nervous picking of skin, biting nails, ticks and changing clothes frequently. If this extreme preoccupation interferes with work, social life, school and general day-to-day functioning it is important to seek help.

If you suspect that your client/patent has BDD you should refer them to someone to rule out other medical conditions or mental health problems. This needs to be done in an appropriate manner which won't cause distress to the client/patient. They may also just go somewhere else and never receive the help that they really need. A psychological assessment can be undertaken to assess risk factors, feelings and behaviours associated with negative self-image and provide a diagnosis of BDD.

From there the person can receive appropriate treatment to help them live the best

life they can without unnecessarily harming themselves by undertaking too many

procedures.

TASK:- Have a look at some people who are suspected of having BDD. The Riverdale star Lili Reinhart. Pete Burns. Jackie Stalone. Karen Carpenter. Amy Winehouse. Shauna Sand. Lolo Ferrari. Joan Van Ark. Katie Price. Latoya and Michael Jackson (family history).

See if you can find any more, and watch some YouTube documentaries,

especially if you are undertaking Phlebotomy training in order to perform it in an

Aesthetic clinic.

S.O.A.P.E.

When we do consultations we commonly use this acronym which stands for;

S = Subjective statement by the client/patient. You should always write exactly what they say, with no exceptions. Must be in their exact words as this is a legal document. This is what they feel is wrong, needs to be done, or concerns they have etc.

O = Objective statement by you the professional practitioner. This will be your statement on what you have assessed and make a summary of your findings or conclusions. (e.g. a health and beauty diagnosis may be in beauty a skin analysis. In health say foot health may be a biomechanics or neuromuscular assessment etc).

A = Action. What service or procedure are you good to recommend for the condition diagnosed? This can be split into short-term actions right now. Long-term action, a few days, weeks, months later etc, and forms part of the plan.

P = Plan. In the plan, you will agree on this in cooperation with your client/patient and in accordance with accepted standards for the procedure. For example, in beauty, the client may need a number of treatments to obtain a certain result. In health, it may be the same. They may need to attend certain treatments on certain days at certain times for them to achieve their goal

E = Evaluation. Evaluation is important. As a hospital phlebotomist this probably won't be a big part of your job, apart from evaluating the immediate effects of the procedure. However, if you're going to offer Phlebotomy in private practice for certain things such as treatments for Iron Overload (Haemochromatosis).

You will need to undertake the evaluation of blood test results to see if your patient requires a bloodletting treatment.

You undertake the evaluation of what has previously been done, and what is left to do, or monitor to make changes to treatment plans accordingly. This helps you make adaptations and changes as appropriate.

PHOTOGRAPHY

Unless you are undertaking Phlebotomy for beauty or aesthetic purposes you won't need to take this aspect into account. Remember if you take photographs for whatever purpose e.g. baseline for treatments and to check responses. You must obtain the client's written consent to do so, and keep the stored in an appropriately secure place.

For example on a computer that is password protected and only accessible to you. To promote privacy and confidentiality, and adherence to the data protection act.

NOTES, ADMIN & MANAGEMENT

A professional practitioner will always keep up-to-date notes and complete admin as they go. As we've mentioned before records, notes, and admin is important so that other practitioner who may come along and treat that client/patient can see everything that has been done before and the current treatment plan agreed. But also because these notes and records are legal documents.

We live in an increasingly litigious society where people will sue you for anything. So you need to be vigilant and keep your notes accurate, and administration up to date. Because you never know when you may need to submit them as evidence to insurers or even courts.

The onus of proof is on the client/patient to prove that you were negligent. If you adhere to accepted protocols and keep accurate legal notes and records you will be able to prove that you have looked after your client/patient as best you can.

Sometimes clients/patients will not complete things on consultation forms or just conveniently forget to remember that they have a certain condition because they have been told somewhere else they are precluded from treatment. So when they come to you and fill in the forms, they don't tell you. If this is the case and you have the documentary evidence in your possession that they never told you they had something that would preclude them from treatment, just so they could get it.

Then they lied and it's not your fault. This happens many many times, and this is why it's so important to keep proper forms, contracts, photos, notes, records etc. As it is all evidence to help you assess and prove that you did everything legally and lawfully to protect your client/patient.

You may also be required to undertake risk assessments, clinical audits, evaluations, inspections and complete a range of documentation to prove that you have done so. Cleaning rotas.

Sterilisation records etc are all examples of documents you may need to keep in your practice.

An easy way to manage most of the things you need to stay safe and legal is to buy a folder and divide it into sections as I did. I have nine sections in it which cover everything I need.

Yours may be slightly different as tailored to your needs. It should be kept somewhere where everyone that works there can have access to it should they need to find information quickly.

Section 1, Health and safety induction records.

Section 2, Accident report forms.

Section 3, Sterilising and autoclave records.

Section 4, Fire safety and inspection records.

Section 5, Reporting equipment failures, repairs and electrical safety Eg. PAT tests.

Section 6, Statutory clinical waste disposal records and certificates.

Section 7, Environmental management and infection control records. E.g. Audit. Cleaning rotas.

Section 8, Health and safety risk assessments, infection control policies and procedures.

Section 9, Health and safety data sheets, equipment manuals, certificates and insurances.

CUSTOMER SERVICE

No matter what business you're in, you need to build up rapport and trust by being honest, open and knowledgeable. Your client/patient is paying for your expertise and for an unforgettable positive experience.

If you provide this and more they will keep coming back, they will also tell their family and friends, so your business will automatically expand. You must ensure that you treat everyone the same, and give them all the same great customer service experience.

It only takes one bad experience for people to start to bring you down.

Remember that people will usually be quicker to tell their family and friends about bad experiences. It takes them longer to tell them about all the good experiences.

Customer service starts from the very first contact, whether it be by telephone, email etc you should always strive to present a professional demeanour. Answer in a timely manner, and provide help and information so that they can get themselves booked in.

Always have a professional appearance, be clean, and tidy, and keep your work area clean and organised. This tells the client/patient an important message. that you are highly organised and professional.

Always strive to resolve matters simply, timely and leave your client/ patient feeling important and listened too. It's nice to be nice. So if you're nice, your client/patient mirrors you, and will be nice too.

A client/patient who is annoyed about something just wants to be heard, and someone to be nice to them. Again if you do this, they will quickly mirror you and leave feeling happy. Many disputes can be resolved simply by listening and spending time with clients/patients explaining things, and agreeing on a way to move forward that benefits you both.

There may be times when you simply don't want to interact or accept a client/patient. Maybe they were inappropriate, you heard something they said or did that made you feel uncomfortable.

It's completely ok to refuse to treat them, especially if you feel unsafe. Just tell them you can't see them. You don't owe them any explanations. If you are employed in a hospital and a similar thing happens you should always seek the advice of your supervisor. They will probably get someone else to take over.

BY NICKY PEARCE

HEALTH AND SAFETY LAWS (UK)

In the UK our current health and safety laws are made up from many different statutes or acts which have been developed over the previous hundred and fifty years of British industrial experience and prompted by serious incidents in the past. If you live in a different country you may also have similar laws, so you need to check them out and see which ones apply to you.

Every person in the workplace whether it be a clinic, or even your home has a duty of care for the health and safety of yourself, any colleagues that may work with or for you, and also the clients/patients who visit you for services.

These basic health and safety laws are there to help you perform appropriate risk assessments and audits so that you can evaluate, monitor and manage any potential risks to you, your colleagues or clients/patients.

If you don't do this you will leave yourself open to problems which may lead to prosecution, bad reputation and even closure of your business. The last thing you want is a criminal record or even time in jail.

In the UK the best place to find information on all relevant laws to you is your local health and safety executive (HSE) from your local council. Some laws are national and some are local to your particular council.

This comes under the local government miscellaneous act, which allows local councils to set additional standards or requirements e.g. licensure. This is why you should always check the local requirements where you live (UK), because one council might have a slightly different law than another. E.G. In my home town of Northwich, our council didn't require Electrologists to register, whereas in Blackpool they did. The reason was that at that time Northwich had no incidence of HIV or hepatitis where as Blackpool did.

It's always worth sending your local HSE an email just to check and keep the email as a record of communication so that you can prove you asked.

Depending on the service, if you just open up you may well receive a visit from the HSE, where they may shut you down until you have received your license etc.

In the UK the Health and Safety at Work Act 1974, is the main act which incorporates earlier legislation including the **Offices, Shops and Railway Premises Act 1963, and the Fire Precautions Act 1971.**

It defines the basic standards which are required in the different types of workplaces.

Employers and employees' responsibilities. The local HSE appoint inspectors who are called Environmental Health Officers (EHO's), and they inspect and enforce the laws.

This act and subsequently the **Workplace (Health, Safety and Welfare) regulations 1992.** Covers aspects of safety regarding;

Maintenance of workplace and equipment.

Ventilation.

Temperature.

(Minimum temperature should be 16oC, but not too warm as to cause risk of heat stroke).

Lighting. (Adequate lighting to do jobs and for safety).

Cleanliness and correct hygiene and disposal of hazardous or clinical waste materials.

Layouts regarding doors, exits, windows and traffic routes. Safe floors, falls and falling objects. Escalators and moving walkways etc.

As a future employer, if you decide to open your own practice, you will be required to have a written health and safety policy and procedures.

This used to be if you had 5 or more employees, but this has changed as you will note later on. Therefore this loophole has now been closed. An employer will have to display certain posters for employees within the workplace so that they can refer to them.

These policies and procedures should also have details of chemicals used in the workplace e.g. in an appropriate locked metal cupboard, stock or dispensaries etc which come under the

Control of Substances Hazardous to Health (COSHH) regulations 2002.

Under COSHH regulations employers have to display posters and mandatory signs.

Policies and procedures should be updated and employees' attention drawn to any changes on a regular basis, so as to keep up to date.

When we have new employees or students on a clinical placement, one of the first things we do with them is to give them an induction.

During the induction, we show them everything that they need to know about safety. Where to find the health and safety folder. COSHH cupboard. First Aider, first aid box and accident report forms. The cleaning & sterilisation process.

Security procedures.

What to do in the event of a fire, and what documentation they need to complete for tasks as appropriate.

Employees have a responsibility to report hazards to the appropriate person, so that correct action can be taken immediately, so as to prevent anyone from getting harmed. Therefore rubbish or obstacles blocking stairs or exits should be reported. Spillages and electrical or equipment failures were reported as well.

BY NICKY PEARCE

In 1992 the European Union updated new legislation which now covers fewer than 5 employees, and is called the Management of Health and Safety at Work Regulations 1999 and is still in force even though Britain has left the E.U.

This relatively new piece of legislation closed the loophole that didn't require any rules for 5 or fewer people. So all health and safety laws apply now.

The Personal Protective Equipment (PPE) at Work Regulations of 1992, requires managers to assess practices via risk assessments to see if PPE is needed in order to undertake work safely.

For example when you use a substance to clean with. On the COSHH health and safety data sheet it may state that you're required to wear gloves or closed shoes and be trained in how to mix and use different things safely.

Employers should provide appropriate PPE for their employees, in order to do their job safely e.g. gloves, aprons, goggles, masks, and alcohol gels.

For some of you dealing with potentially infectious body fluids, you will need to use standard precautions when treating people as you do not know what they may be carrying. You can't tell if someone is carrying an infectious disease, especially if you're the one taking the blood from them to test in the lab, so you should just assume everyone has one and use standard precautions.

One of the most important things to do to help reduce the risk of cross-infection is to wash your hands before and after contact with clients/patients. Use gloves if appropriate and or alcohol based hand gels.

When manual handling the Manual Handling and Lifting Operations Regulations 1992 come into play.

Most occupations involve some aspect of manual handling and lifting so risk assessments should be carried out taking this into account. Risk of injury. The manual movement involved in the activity. The physical constraint the activity involves. The environmental constraints imposed by the work environment. Workers' individual capabilities. Actions to be taken to minimise potential risks. In clinical environments, you will receive approved training.

You should always bend your knees not your back. Never lift any more than you can comfortably. Get help if needed. Carry the heaviest part of something closest to you. Don't carry any more than 4 kg or 2 kg split into each arm so as to balance equally.

Provision and Use of Work Equipment Regulations (PUWER) 1998. Lays down the regulations regards the selection and safe use of workplace equipment. E.G. training required to operate equipment, testing, location and installation maintenance.

Health ad Safety (Display Screen Equipment) Regulations 1992. Specify the safe levels of radiation acceptable from computer screens, and define safe sitting distances, screen filters, breaks from usage to prevent eye strain and headaches etc.

BY NICKY PEARCE

Control of Substances Hazardous to Health (COSHH) regulations 2002.

As previously discussed COSHH regulations are there to help employers protect the workplace and prevent injury to eyes, skin, inhalation etc. From hazardous substances which are regularly used in the workplace.

Each substance should come with a health and safety data sheet, which details its composition, correct storage, and any first aid measures. Risk assessments need to be done so that potential risks whilst being used can be identified, minimised or eliminated.

Chemicals come with symbols on the side which should be noted.

Staff that use these products should be fully trained in their safe usage. All chemicals should be stored in a lockable, explosive-proof metal cabinet when not in use.

Health and Safety (First Aid) Regulations 1981.

It is recommended that each workplace have at least 1 HSE qualified First Aider. Or someone with appropriate First Aid training. All employees should be informed preferably at induction who is the designated First Aider, and where to locate the first aid box. First Aid kits are made to cover the appropriate number of people in the workplace. The accident book or accident form should be completed after such an event.

All accidents occurring in the workplace must be reported and commented on in the accident book or accident report form.

Reporting of Injuries, Diseases and Dangerous Occurrences Regulations (RIDDOR) 1995.

In certain circumstances, it is a legal requirement that you report these things if they happen to employees, trainees or visitors to the local enforcement officer in writing. These circumstances are; Loss of sight. Amputation. Fracture. Electric shock. When an occurrence causes death, major injury or a stay in a hospital of more than 24 hours.

You must contact the enforcement officer first by telephone and then a written report sent within 7 days. This must be documented in the accident book and kept for a minimum of 3 years from that date for the HSE to inspect should they need to investigate.

TASK:- Look online for chemical symbols used on products then look through your cupboards at home to identify the dangers. You may come across many of these symbols in your lab at work.

BY NICKY PEARCE

Clinical Waste Management:

This is covered in the UK by various acts e.g.

The Environmental Protection Act 1990. This is the main legislation which governs clinical waste disposal. (Including duty of care regulations). It states that all producers of waste have a duty of care to ensure the correct management of waste, including documenting the transfer of waste and ensuring waste is handled correctly. It also requires compliance with waste Hierachy.

The Controlled Waste Regulations 2012 (England and Wales). This states that household, industrial and commercial waste is classed as "CONTROLLED WASTE" and is subject the the

Environmental Protection Act 1990.

The Hazardous Waste Directive 2005. This provides guidance on labelling, record keeping, monitoring and control obligations for everyone from waste production to final recovery and disposal. It forbids the mixing of hazardous substances and items in order to prevent risk to the environment and human health.

In Scotland, we have the Scottish Environmental Protection Agency.

When producing clinical waste you must have it collected and disposed of according to the law by a registered clinical waste company.

When you call them they will ask you some questions about the kind of clinical waste you have so they can complete an audit. They will send you the audit and you should print it and keep it safe. They will then send you appropriate receptacles e.g. clinical waste bins, sharps bins, and bags of various colours depending on the clinical waste you generate.

You must ensure the correct waste goes into the correct receptacle. When they pick it up they will provide you with a waste transfer certificate and a certificate of destruction. You must keep these documents safe for a minimum of 3 years just in case they are needed to be checked by the HSE inspectors.

Fire Precautions Act 1971. States that all staff must be trained on fire evacuation procedures.

This is done at induction remember. Emergency exits must be signposted and meeting places designated so that everyone can be accounted for. A fire safety certificate is required from the fire brigade if there are more than 20 employees on the premises or more than 10 employees on different floors.

INSURANCE (UK).

With regards to the workplace, there is only one compulsory insurance that an employer must have and that's **Employers Liability Insurance.**

This policy provides financial compensation to employees should they have an account at work. This certificate must be displayed at the workplace.

Other forms of insurance are a good idea, and these are;

Public Liability Insurance protects the employer and employees against claims made in the event of an accident or death of a third party on the premises e.g. a client trips, falls or dies because something falls on them for example.

Professional Indemnity Insurance extends Public Liability Insurance to cover in the event a claim is made against a particular employee.

Product and Treatment Liability Insurance is usually included with your Public Liability insurance but should be checked to make sure. Product Liability Insurance protects you against claims made by clients/patients if you prescribe, use or sell the wrong product.

There are many types of insurance you may wish to consider, an insurance broker will be able to provide help, information and costs.

Some businesses also go for Business Interruption Insurance. Should you have to close down for one reason, you would be paid for being out of business.

BASIC MEDICAL MICROBIOLOGY AND PUBLIC HEALTH

To be effective at infection control you must know a little about the micro-organisms which cause pathological disease in humans and how to disrupt its transmission through cleaning, good health promotion and education to improve immune function and use of standard precautions and sterile techniques to block portals of entry into the body.

It's a good idea to have a checklist of cleaning, PPE and other procedures and products you need to do at the beginning, the end of every day, and in between each client/patient. You will soon do this automatically and not need the checklist.

If you are starting your own business you should design a cleaning rota and keep it up to date by signing and dating it. Keep this in your folder to track and manage your infection control measures.

Hygiene and management of cross-infection is essential when performing for example phlebotomy or microneedling. We use hygienic procedures and products to disrupt portals of entry into patients' micro-organisms which can cause diseases.

There are many classes of micro-organisms which can cause disease in humans, and some can cross over from animal to human as well.

BY NICKY PEARCE

The most common ones are;

Bacteria or single-celled (Eukaryotic before nucleus) micro-organisms. Some medically important ones are Streptococcus and Staphylococcus.

Viruses, the most important ones to be aware of here are mainly Blood Bournes Viruses or BBV's

Hepatitis, of which there are a few species the most important being A, B & C. Human Immune Deficiency Virus HIV.

Bacteria can be treated using antibiotics, Viruses on the other hand are more difficult to treat, for example, hepatitis can be treated with antivirals or vaccinations.

I would always recommend getting vaccinated for both Hepatitis A & B especially when undertaking a healthcare job for self-protection.

You can speak to your family doctor about getting these. HIV is treated using antivirals which suppress its replication but don't eradicate it. HIV patients who take regular meds will become undetectable and their life expectancy is the same as anyone else nowadays. HIV is treated like any other chronic disease with meds and people with HIV normally die from old age or age-related illnesses like everyone else.

There are also fungal infections, Protozoal infections and Prion infections, but you will rarely come into contact with these.

Left untreated many infectious diseases can be debilitating and even cause serious injury and death. So you can see why it's important to have a basic understanding of the main ones and why you should always adhere to hygiene procedures.

Adhering to hygiene procedures and keeping everything clean and sterile, protects you and your patients from cross-infection, or the transference of one infection to another person.

There are a number of ways in which you can do this.

1. Clean your equipment regularly.

2. Use only sterile, pre-packed and single-use items. Dispose of them immediately into an approved sharps container.

3. Use standard precautions e.g. PPE Gloves, Apron, Goggles, Masks etc especially if taking samples from patients with infectious diseases. The medical staff will alert you as to what PPE is required. But your basic PPE is Gloves and an apron.

4. The most effective thing you can do to prevent cross-infection is to wash your hands before and after any contact with each patient. Find the hand washing song online and practice washing your hands.

Don't EVER underestimate the effectiveness of hand washing for controlling cross infection. Your hands are germ factories, you touch doors, beds, and other foamites constantly which other people have touched and may have transferred micro-organisms onto them.

You are accountable, so you may be required to document the cleaning and hygiene procedures you have undertaken where appropriate and keep a record of these measures you have taken to reduce the likelihood of cross-infection.

Before using any cleanser on your patient always check and ask them if they are allergic to anything. Some patients may be allergic to latex gloves, so use nitrile instead. Some may be allergic to chlorhexidine so don't use anything with that in. Just ask, or if you can't then check with the nurse or doctor beforehand.

If in a hospital it may be posted behind the bed or in the patient notes at the foot of the bed, you can check the allergies section first.

Occupational health or A&E. WATCH THE NEEDLESTICK INJURY VIDEO.at our YouTube "Nicky Pearce".

CONTRA-INDICATIONS. CONTRA-ACTIONS (HEALING CRISIS). AFTERCARE.

There are two types of contra-indications. Absolute where you would definitely not undertake a procedure if a client/patient had one of the designated conditions. relative, where you would maybe modify the procedure and adapt it to make it safer for the client/patient.

With each treatment or procedure, there will be a list of absolute and relative contra-indications to which you must adhere to.

Contra-actions are also called healing crises. They are common reactions to procedures which you must tell your client/patient about, otherwise you risk inadvertently stressing them out.

This is also why aftercare is so important. You must provide both verbal and written aftercare advice to your client/patient. You should always aim to go through these contra-actions (healing crises) and aftercare advice before you even start a procedure. Then afterwards go over them again and provide a leaflet. You can design your own leaflet to give them so that they can refer back to it should they need reassurance.

Always document that you have given both verbal and written aftercare in the client's notes and get them to sign that they have received it. Again this is to protect you as a practitioner legally as well.

CONSENT

Clients/patients must sign to give their explicit consent to having a treatment done by practitioners. This consent should only be taken off the back of informed consent, where the client/patient has had all their questions answered fully. They have discussed risks, benefits, features, potential outcomes and you have managed their expectations appropriately.

The practitioner signs to say that he is satisfied with the client/patients decision.

For all forms to become legal documents they must be signed and dated appropriately.

Clients are obliged to give you accurate information so that you can provide appropriate, and safe treatments to them.

Implicit consent is given when for example if you're going to take someone's blood they present and give you their arm.

Both kinds of consent can be removed by either party at any time.

In the UK you are legally required to keep records for a minimum of 7 years from the last date a client/patient attended. You must then destroy them in accordance with the law.

The Data Protection Act 1998.

Requires some businesses in the UK that keep information about others either on forms or computers etc, to register with the information control officer.

There is usually an annual fee, and you can go online and answer a quick questionnaire to see if you need to be registered. You should always keep records in a secure place.

Paper records should be locked away and computer records protected by passwords and only appropriate staff allowed access. You have a professional, ethical and legal duty to keep client/patient records private and confidential at all times, and never discuss treatments with anyone who is not directly involved with their treatments.

You should also be aware that clients/patient have a right to see their records at any time and you should provide access and or copies if asked to. So as mentioned previously, be careful what you write and keep the language professional and accurate.

REFLECTIVE PRACTICE

Reflective practice is another way to develop your professional skills through your thought processes. Reflective practice can take place at any time.

You can either just simply sit there and reflect on a situation that has occurred, or you can write it down as part of a reflective practice diary.

Reflection is a very important part of professional life and we all do it. It can form part of your continual professional development if you document it.

Reflective practice is a process which enables you to achieve a better understanding of yourself, your skills, competencies, knowledge, any gaps, and professional practice. It is useful to document reflection because we can go back and read through it to identify how we process events. Evaluate our experiences, thoughts, feelings and understand relevant issues which might pop up.

The objective is to identify what we have and haven't learnt in order to construct a plan to try new approaches to learning from mistakes, or as the case may be keep doing something because it worked out well.

We can enhance future practice, or recognise and validate effectively practice to utilise in the future.

Learning comes from nay different incidents and experiences that we have in life. We can learn much about ourselves, others, our job, our organisation, interactions with different people, skills and abilities if we critically analyse them appropriately, It's a cycle of events check out (Gibs Reflective Cycle 1988).

GIBBS REFLECTION CYCLE

It starts with; Describe what happened.

Feelings (what were you thinking)?

What was good and bad about the experience?

What sense can you make of the situation?

Analysis?

Conclusion (What else could you have done)?

Evaluation.

Action plan (If it arose again what would you do)?

Then back to the start with; Describe what happened. When it happens again to see what happened this time. Did you implement anything from the action plan?

BUSINESS

You are probably undertaking this course to either start a new business or extend your scope of practice. Business is another subject that isn't usually taught in courses, so I will quickly point you in the right direction to study relevant subjects that you will definitely need to avail yourself of.

One of the best ways to start to think about business is to go online to a major bank website and look on their page for a business plan template. You can download this and start to think about filling it in.

BY NICKY PEARCE

Business planning is an essential part of owning and running a successful business. A business plan needs to be fluid and adaptable according to your requirements and the market.

Think about business and how they had to adapt to survive during the recent pandemic for example. A lot of businesses closed down because they weren't allowed to open, but a lot of businesses found a way to take their products and services online. So they stayed afloat and survived. This is why you have to be one step ahead of your game and competition.

Doing the necessary research in order to complete your business plan will give you the skills and knowledge to be able to analyse what's currently going on, and then you can steer your business in the right direction. It makes you focus and get things straight in your mind.

What you want to do, where you want to go, and eventually how you're going to get there.

You may even wish to take out a business loan from a bank, or other backers, to help you start your business, and banks will require a full business plan so that they can assess if you have done your research and know what you are talking about before they decide if you're a good risk to lend money too.

Sections you will commonly find in a business plan are the Mission, a summary of products or services. Market research involves an analysis f the competition, and your competitive edge.

BUSINESS PLANNING CONTINUED

Pricing. Location. Geographical demand for your product or service. Costings and cash flow forecasts. Marketing and promotional plans. Websites, leaflets, brochures, branding etc. Legal obligations e.g. licensure, insurance, accounting, health and safety etc.

Students often look at the size and depth of the research and knowledge required to complete a business plan, as you have to be a jack of all trades, they have to become a good business person, but it's worth putting in the hours at the beginning, as most businesses that don't will fail within the first year of trading.

Undertaking the research, designing things, and branding can and should be fun. You send out your intentions to the universe which will manifest, and begin to attract what you want.

If you can do all this, stay informed and ahead of the competition, then your business will flourish.

You not only need to be good at your profession, but you need to also be good in business as well in order to succeed.

CARDIOVASCULAR SYSTEM ANATOMY AND PHYSIOLOGY

As a Phlebotomist, you will be taking blood samples from the patient's veins so you'll need to know some basics about blood and the cardiovascular system or circulatory system.

The cardiovascular system is made of three basic elements.

The heart or pump.

The delivery tubes or blood vessels e.g. arteries, veins and capillaries, and the blood itself. Blood is one of the body's major transport systems.

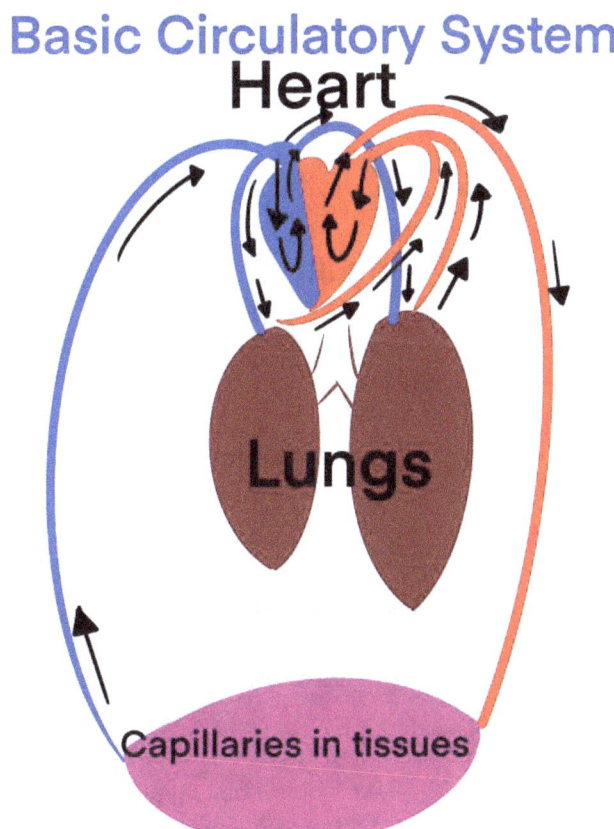

Arteries take oxygenated blood to the tissues and organs. Veins return the blood back to the heart where it's pumped back to the lungs to be re-oxygenated and repumped back around the body again.

The blood you'll be sampling is in the veins, and is deoxygenated, and therefore darker than blood in arteries which is oxygenated and bright red.

Blood is a substance with many physiological functions, and can be used for testing and monitoring purposes.

Blood can be split into two main portions. The liquid component is called Plasma which is approximately 55%, and the cellular component which is approximately 45%.

Plasma is 91% water which contains 7% Proteins in the form of Albumin 55% of the 7% which helps maintain blood volume. 38% are Globulins which help with immune function fighting infection. 7% Clotting factor fibrinogen, and 1.5% electrolytes, trace elements, glucose, hormones, vitamins, amino acids, urea, and antibodies.

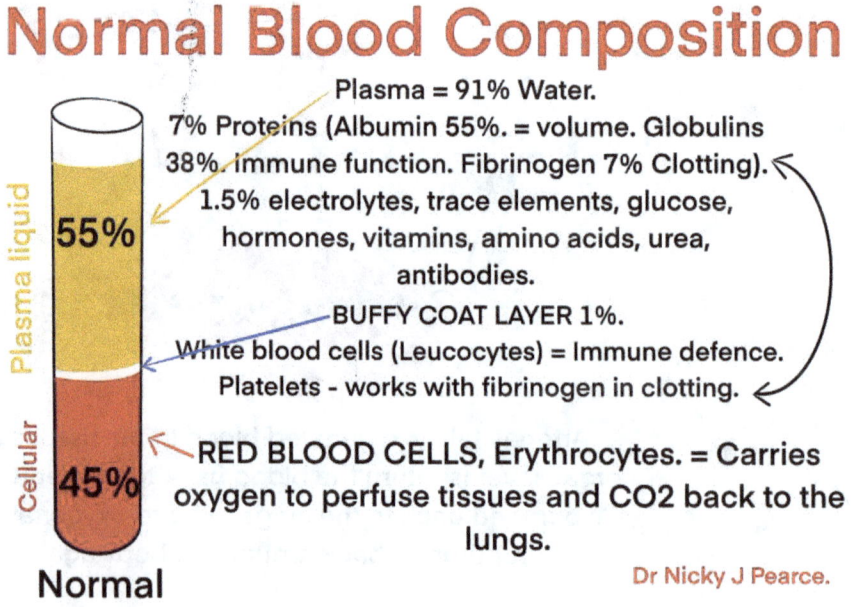

Normal Blood Composition

Plasma = 91% Water.
7% Proteins (Albumin 55%. = volume. Globulins 38%. immune function. Fibrinogen 7% Clotting).
1.5% electrolytes, trace elements, glucose, hormones, vitamins, amino acids, urea, antibodies.
BUFFY COAT LAYER 1%.
White blood cells (Leucocytes) = Immune defence.
Platelets - works with fibrinogen in clotting.
RED BLOOD CELLS, Erythrocytes. = Carries oxygen to perfuse tissues and CO2 back to the lungs.

Dr Nicky J Pearce.

Plasma liquid 55%
Cellular 45%
Normal

BY NICKY PEARCE

When blood is spun or left for an amount of time it separates out and the heaviest or red blood cells sink to the bottom of the plasma and the plasma floats on top.

In between the red blood cells and the plasma is a very thin layer called the Buffy coat layer, which is composed of White Blood Cells or Leucocytes which help with immune response.

This layer also contains platelets, which are special particles of red blood cells which when triggered with clotting factors burst and form clots with fibrinogen like when a scab forms on a cut.

Red Blood Cells or Erythrocytes are specialised cells containing Iron in their Haemoglobin molecules. Haemoglobin picks up oxygen from the lungs and then delivers it to tissues all around the body for cellular respiration.

It also brings back the metabolic waste gas called carbon dioxide or CO_2, and it is diffused and exchanged back into the lungs as oxygen is picked up again.

Therefore CO_2 is exhaled as oxygen is inhaled. This cycle continues throughout life to keep the tissues perfused and oxygenated for life.

Circulatory or breathing changes due to ill health can change the chemistry e.g. acidity of the blood and cause signs and symptoms.

Oxygenated blood is pumped from the heart through larger elastic conducting vessels to medium muscular distributing vessels, which then conduct blood through small arterioles and then capillaries within tissues, and organs of the body.

The oxygen and nutrients are given up to these cells, tissues and organs and waste products from respiration and metabolism is picked up to be transported in the blood to various excreting organs. E.G. Urea is removed by the kidneys, carbon dioxide CO_2 is removed by the lungs, some waste is secreted in sweat and others are transformed in the liver to harmless products which the body can get rid of through the kidneys.

Deoxygenated blood which also contains the waste returns from the capillaries into the small venues, medium veins and larger capacitance or reservoir vessels which lead back into the heart

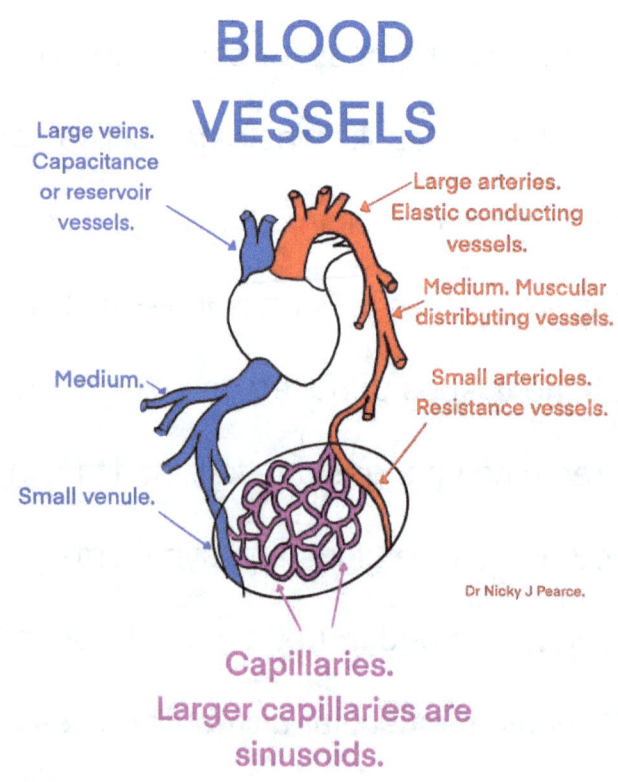

BLOOD VESSELS

Large veins. Capacitance or reservoir vessels.

Large arteries. Elastic conducting vessels.

Medium. Muscular distributing vessels.

Medium.

Small arterioles. Resistance vessels.

Small venule.

Dr Nicky J Pearce.

Capillaries. Larger capillaries are sinusoids.

Arteries are thicker as they contain more layers than veins.

As you can see in these diagrams, the arteries have additional internal and external elastic lamina. This is to aid the heart in pumping the blood around the body and maintaining blood pressure.

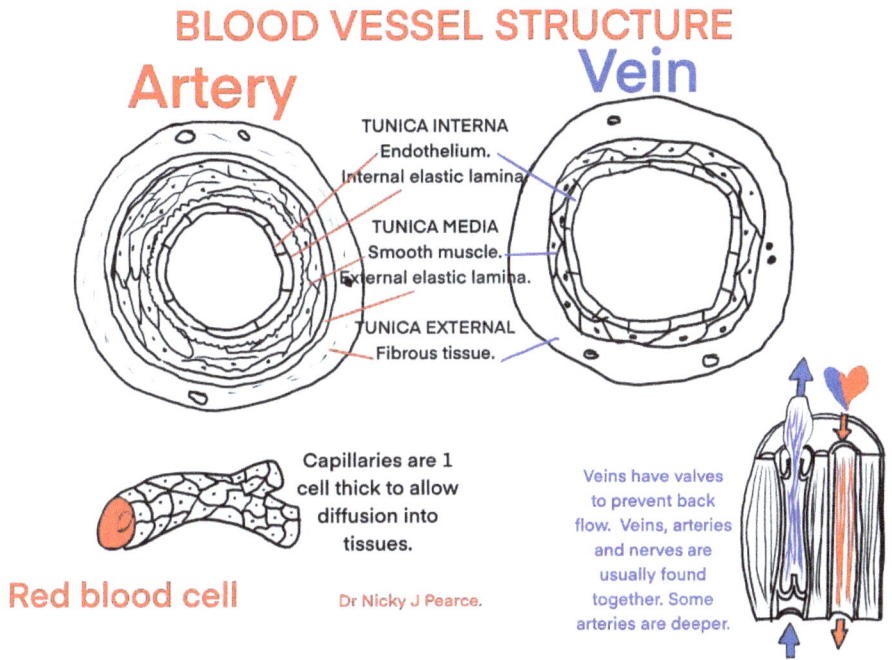

Veins on the other hand only have smooth muscles and valves which help to prevent back flow when blood is pumped back to the heart up the body towards the heart. Muscles which surround veins also help to squeeze the blood back towards the heart. This can be illustrated in the venous foot pump, whereby walking aids in venous return in the foot and leg.

Capillaries are tiny blood vessels one cell thick which help in the transfer or diffusion of oxygen, and nutrients into the tissues and the removal of waste back into the system circulation where it can be gotten rid of by the various detoxifying organs of the body.

THE MAIN VEINS OF THE BODY USED FOR PHLEBOTOMY ARE

Median Cubital vein.   **Cephalic vein.**
Median vein of the forearm.   **Basilic vein.**

This is the order of preference because of the ease of locating them according to

depth and stability.

VEIN ANATOMICAL LOCATIONS

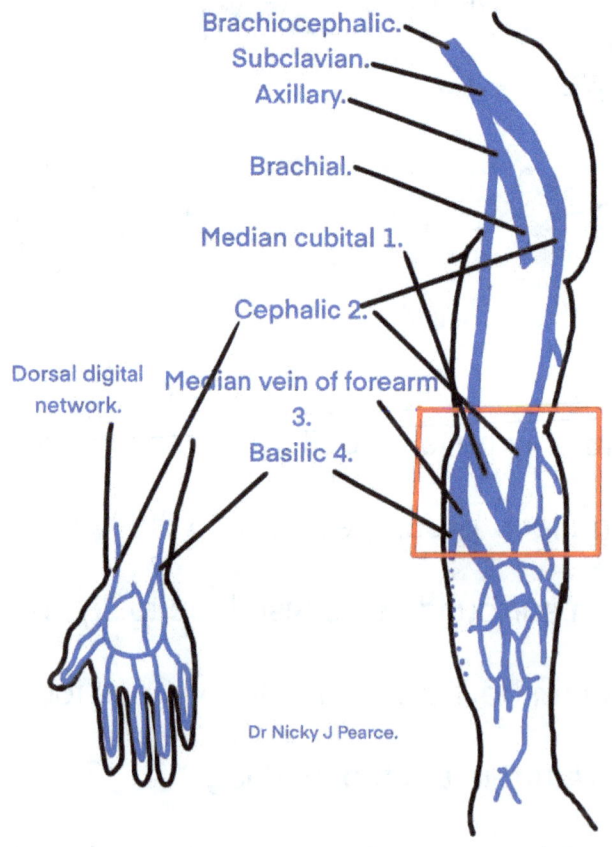

Sometimes the dorsal veins of the hands are used if you are unable to access the

arms.

BY NICKY PEARCE

TIPS FOR ACCESSING BLOOD

Always have the bevel on the needle tip pointing upwards.

Have the needle at an angle of approx 30-45 degrees.

Stabilise the vein by applying tension below it to prevent it from rolling.

Make sure the patient is hydrated and has had their morning tea, coffee, or water.

The nervous patient's veins can collapse.

Reasons blood won't flow......

May not be in the vein. May have passed through. May have missed the vein. May be pushed up against the inside of the vein.

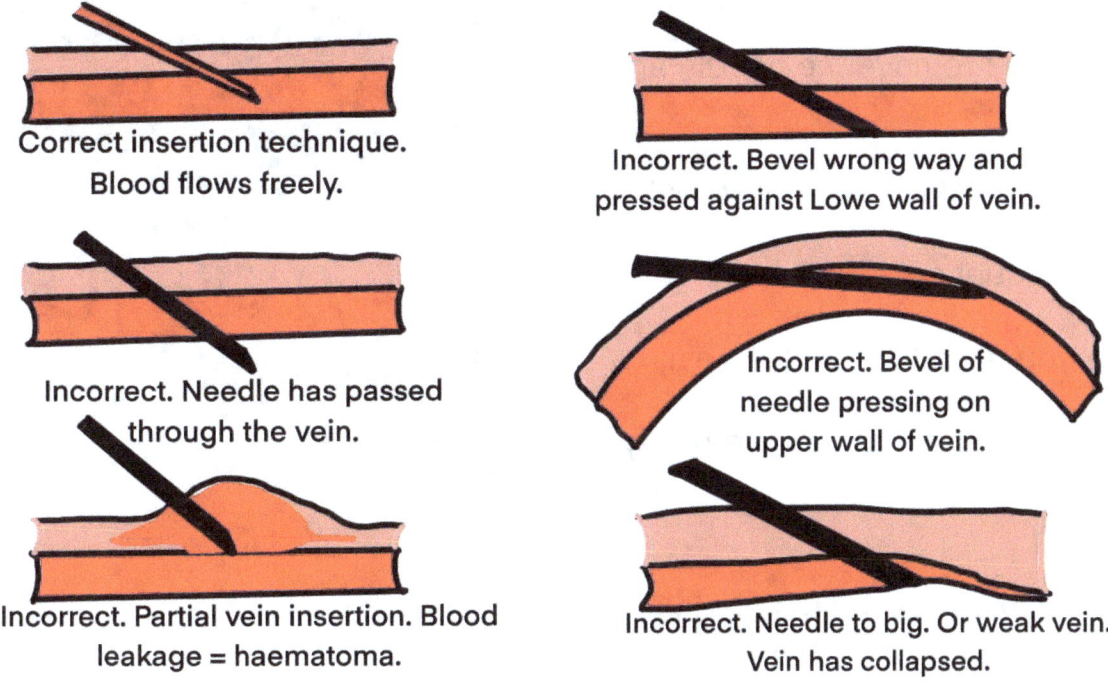

Correct insertion technique.
Blood flows freely.

Incorrect. Bevel wrong way and pressed against Lowe wall of vein.

Incorrect. Needle has passed through the vein.

Incorrect. Bevel of needle pressing on upper wall of vein.

Incorrect. Partial vein insertion. Blood leakage = haematoma.

Incorrect. Needle to big. Or weak vein. Vein has collapsed.

Above are the most common reasons why blood won't flow.

In most needles, there is a window where you can see a flash of blood come up the tube.

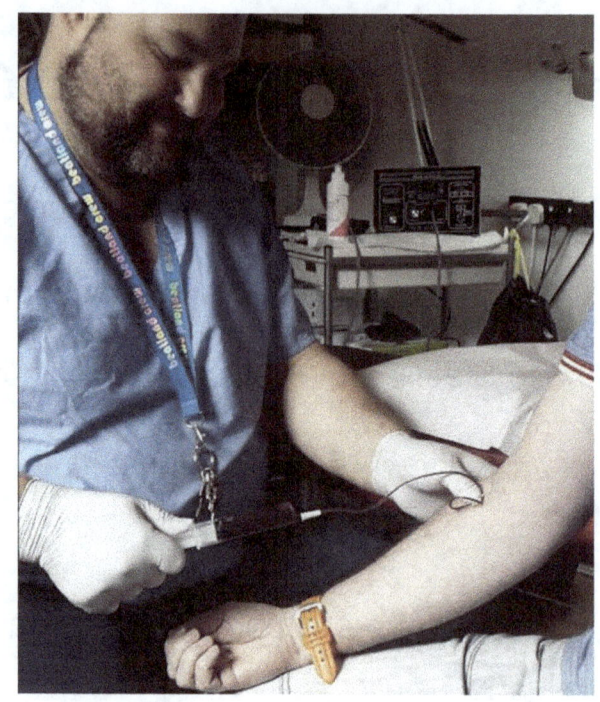

If you suspect you have gone too far in, withdraw the needle slightly and see if this works.

You can adjust your angle slightly and move the point of the needle to relocate.

Don't go digging around, just slight adjustments should work.

If they don't remove the needle and try again.

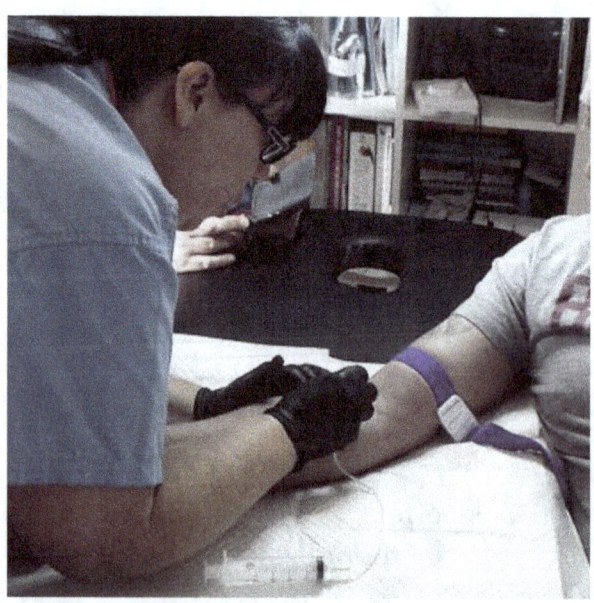

Make sure you palpate the veins whilst you have the tourniquet on.

Once you have located the vein, loosen the tourniquet until you are ready again.

Only apply the tourniquet again when you are ready.

If you use the tourniquet too much it may have an effect on the blood results.

This is called haemoconcentration and may affect Glucose, Potassium, and Cholesterol results.

EQUIPMENT

There's a lot of equipment out there used in the Phlebotomy or Venepunctre practice. The type used will mainly depend on the types of tests to be performed because long tubes can have an effect on blood cells, and the location where you work. They may have particular preferences.

The most important aspect is however that it must be;

STERILE. PRE-PACKED & DISPOSABLE! (With needle covers).

Also in a lot of countries such as the UK, Europe and the USA, it is now a legal requirement to have needles that have automatic retractable or activated mechanisms. This is to prevent the risk of Needle Stick Injuries.

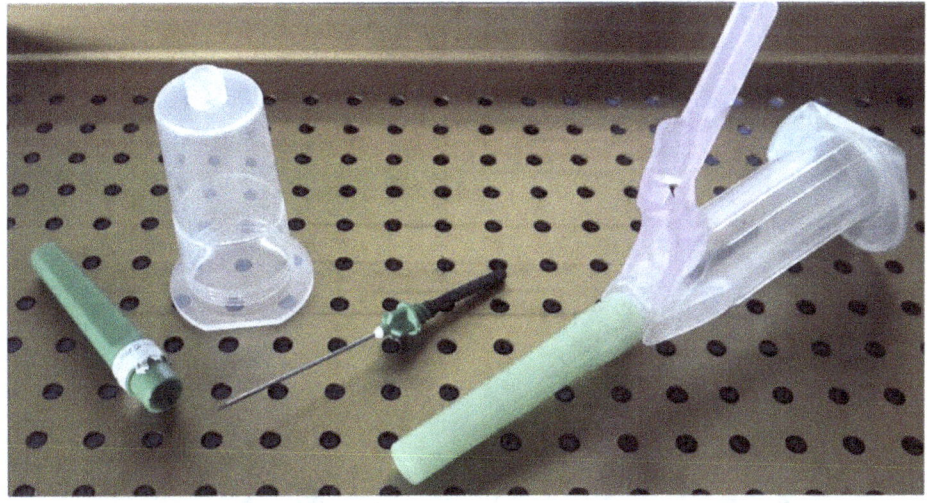

In the photo above; These are needles and tubes that are used in conjunction with pressurised vacutainers.

The needle is inserted into the vein and tubes or vacutainers are inserted into the tube which has a needle on the inside. The needle pierces into the tube and the tube sucks the blood out of the vein.

The needle on the left does not have a cover, whereas the one on the right does. It is activated manually by the Phlebotomist pushing it down and clicking it over the needle.

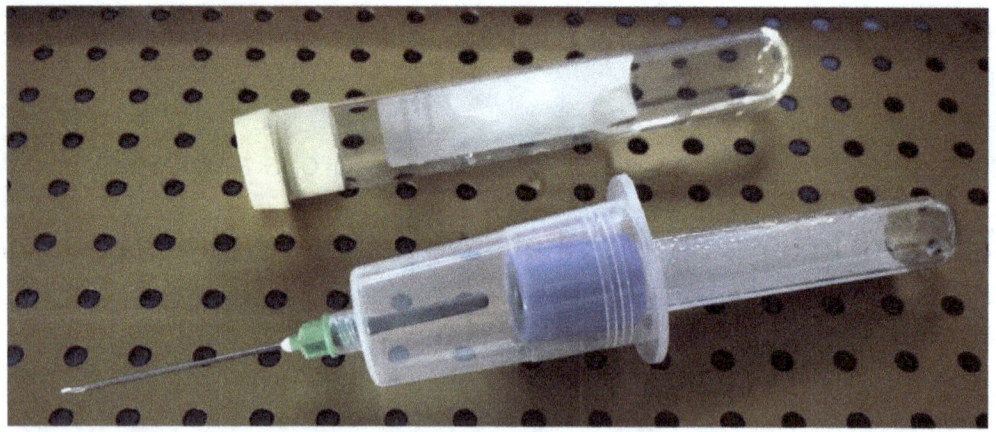

Above is how Vacutainers fit together to work.

NEEDLE AND SYRINGE COMBINATION

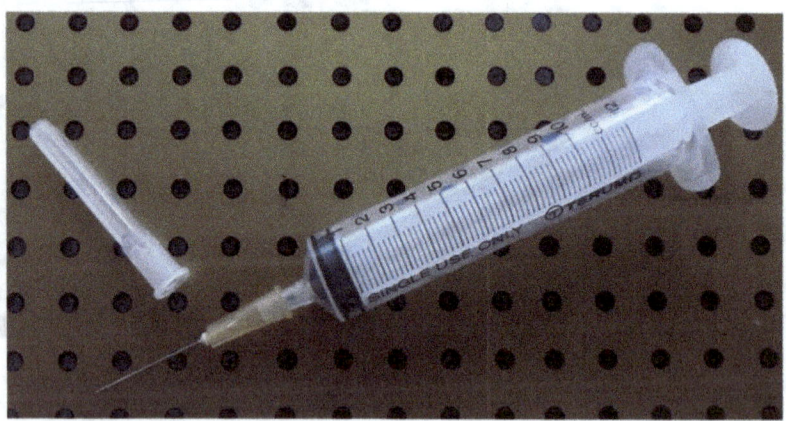

Above is a photo of the traditional set-up of needle and syringe.

BY NICKY PEARCE

Undertaking phlebotomy using the needle and syringe set-up is highly skilled, especially to be safe and avoid needlstick injuries.

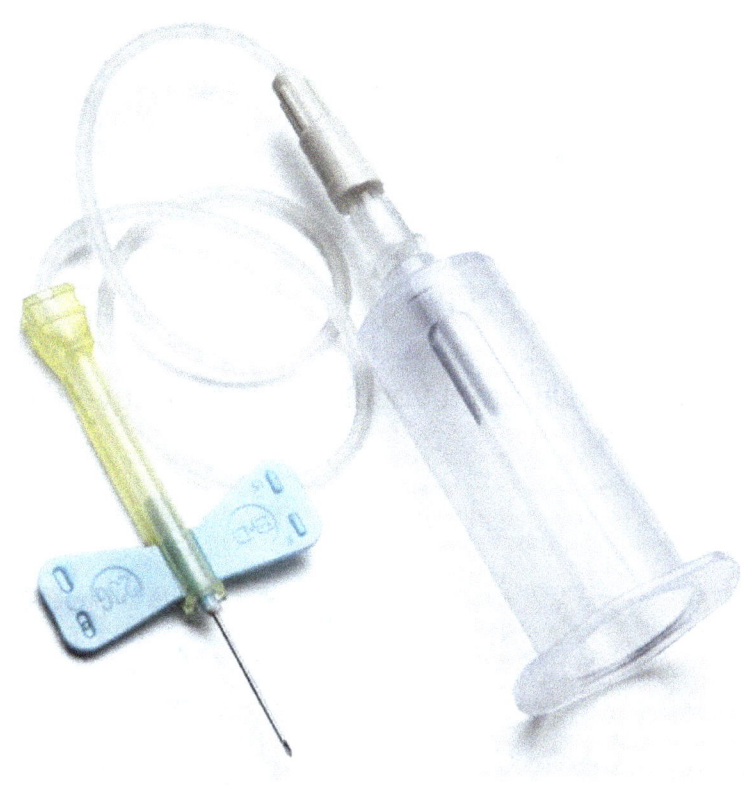

Above is a photo of a butterfly needle with a tube attached to a Vacutainer tube. Alternatively, it can also be attached to a syringe. Butterfly needles also need to have automatic retractable needles or activated needle covers.

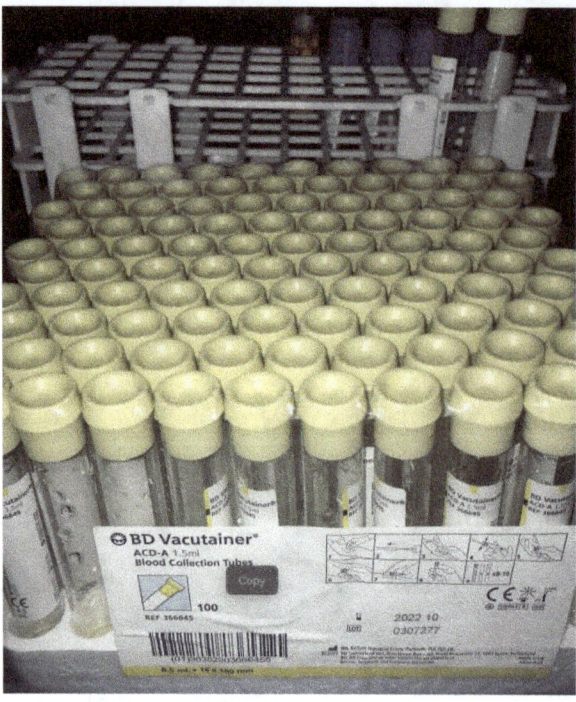

Above photo of vacationers. Different vacutainers may have different additives to work with the blood samples.

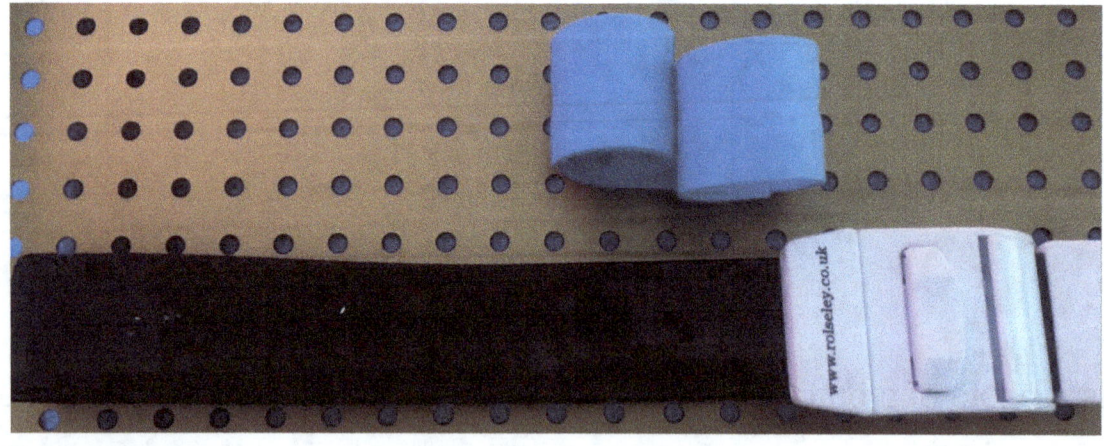

Above is a Blue disposable tourniquet, and a Black non-disposable quick-release tourniquet.

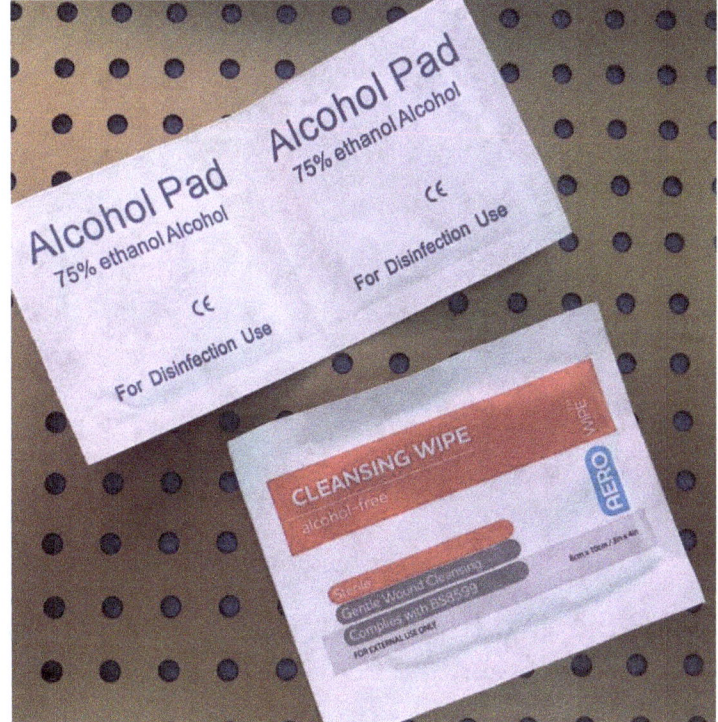

Above is a selection of Alcoholic prep wipes. Use these in circles, starting in one spot and working out. Leave to dry on the skin for at least 90 seconds.

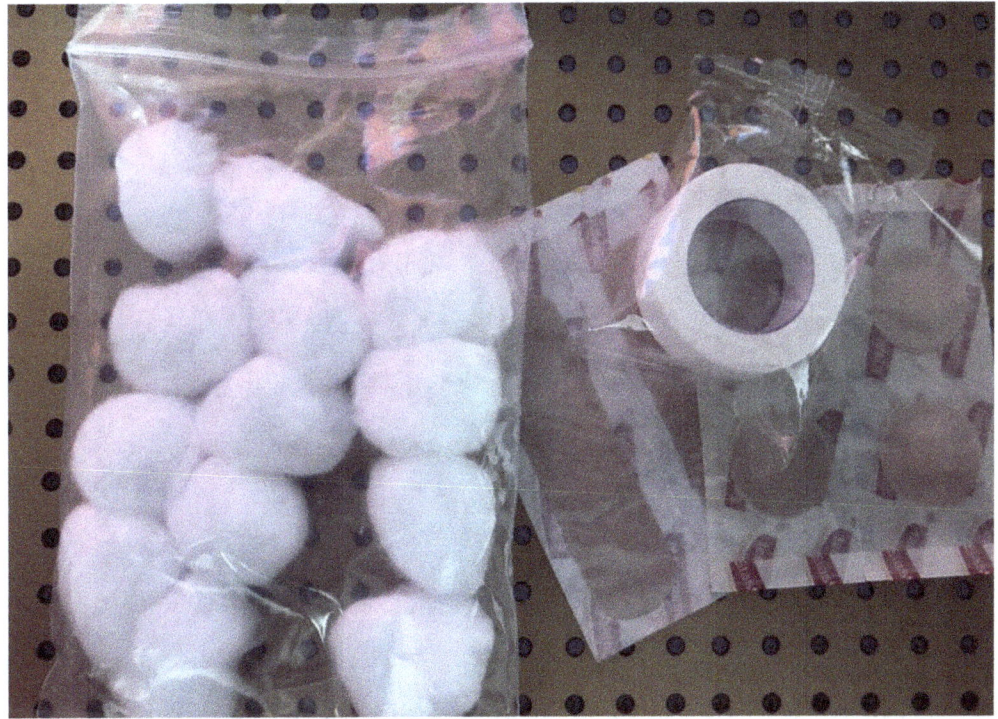

Above a selection of cotton wool, tape or hypoallergenic plasters. to put on the puncture site after the procedure.

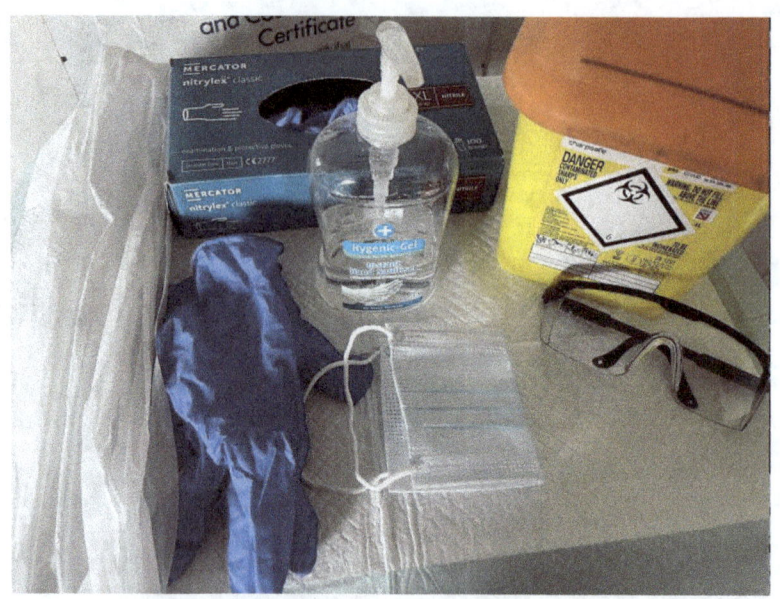

Above is all the Personal Protective Equipment (PPE), that you may require. Apron. Gloves. Alcohol gel. Mask. Goggles & Sharps Box.

DON'T FORGET YOUR FINE-TIPPED MAKRER TO WRITE.

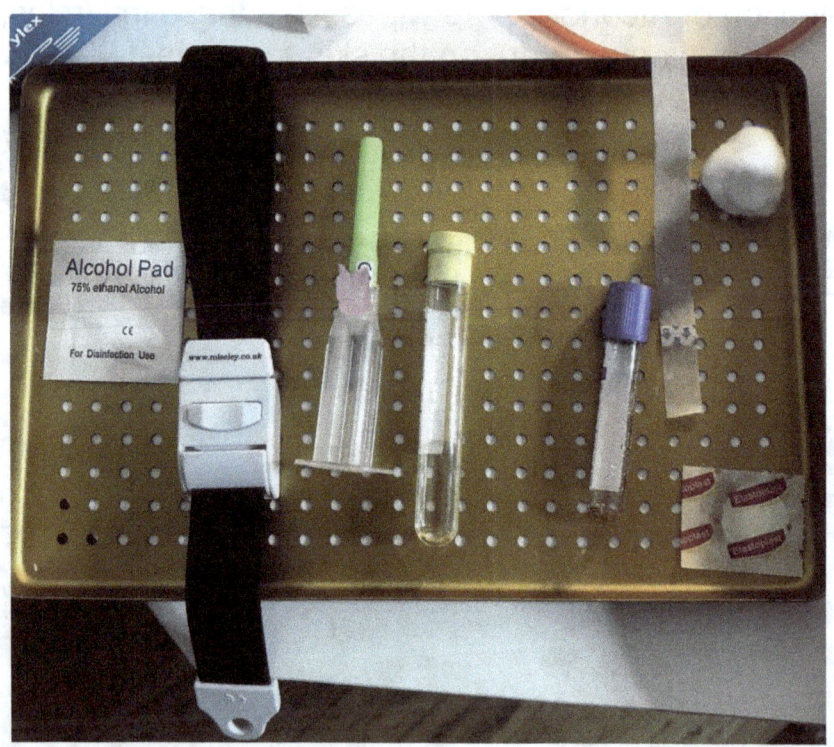

Lay out your equipment and supplies on your tray in the order that you are going to use them.

EXAMPLE; Identity the patient. Consent. Palpate (With or without a tourniquet). Alcohol prep. Re-apply tourniquet. Insert needle, then vacutainers in order. (When you remove vacutainers gently invert to mix blood with contents 5 - 10 times). Release the tourniquet before taking the needle out. Remove the needle and apply pressure and cotton wool. Apply a plaster over the puncture site. Label tubes as per the requirements. Sometimes patient stickers are used. This depends on the policies and procedures.

Check the patient is ok before you leave. Put everything back the way it was before. Let the staff know that you have finished if drips need to be restarted up again.

NEEDLE SIZES AND USES

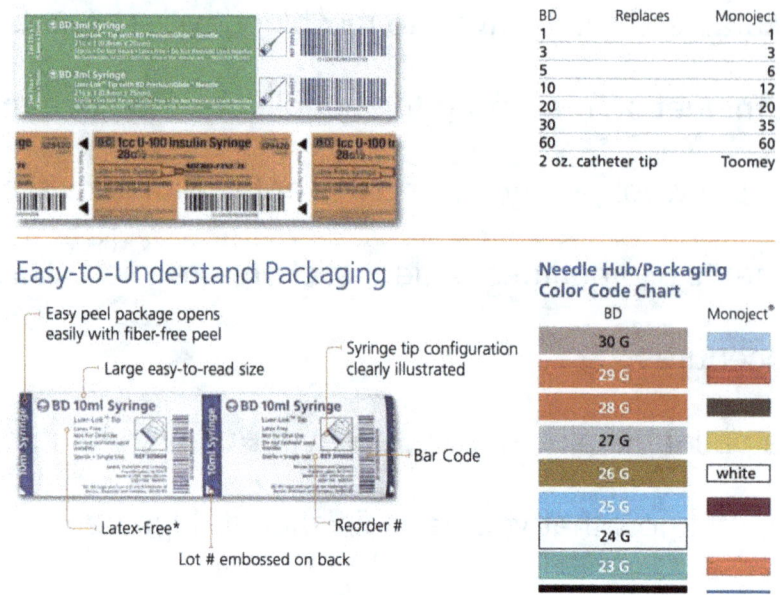

GAUGE	COLOUR	USE
16	WHITE	Mainly used in ICU, blood transfusions where large and rapid amounts of fluids need to be given.
18	PINK	Mainly used for aspiration of fluid from the body or cavity. Also for pushing fluids rapidly e.g, in CT PE protocols or other imaging or testing that requires large IV sizes.
18	RED	Used to draw up medicines.
19	CREAM / IVORY	Used for injecting viscous medicines.
20	YELLOW	Used for both IV and IM injections.
21	GREEN	Used in phlebotomy and also for injecting thicker non water based medications.
22	BLCK	Used for IM injections into superficial muscles where there maybe capillary fragility or bleeding concern.
23	BLUE	Used in phlebotomy for small veins.
24	PURPLE	Used in phlebotomy for small veins.
24	VIOLET	Used for Intradermal, Subcutaneous, Intramuscular, Intravenous injections and aspiration.
25	ORANGE	Used in syringe drivers, TB testing, Allergy testing, Insulin injections, and local anaesthetics.
26	BROWN	Used for IM or IV injections depending on needle length.
27	GREY	Used in subcutaneous injection, and injections into superficial veins in the hands, arms, feet and lower leg.

LABORATORY TESTS

You should familiarise yourself with the Departments and tests that they do. This will become useful when learning the bottles and order of drawing blood later.

Sometimes multiples of the same bottles may be required because multiple Departments might need the same additives used.

Different Departments might be located in different parts of the hospital as well, so it's useful to give each department a small bottle for themselves so that they don't have to share or go hunting around for samples.

BIOCHEMISTRY

Urea and Electrolytes (U&E's). Creatine, Sodium, Potassium.

C-reactive protein (CRP) for specific inflammation detection. Erythrocyte Sedimentation Rate (ESR) for non-specific inflammation detection.

Amylase assay. Bone profile. Magnesium assay. Iron studies. Lipid profile. Vitamins. Glucose. HBA1c.

Thyroid function tests (TFT's).

Troponins (2 Need to be done, at different times).

Creatine kinase. Urate. Serum osmolality (requires a urine test at the same time as taking blood).

ENDOCRINOLOGY

Beta-hCG. Calcitonin. Cortisol. EPO. Sex hormones. Growth hormone. IGF1. Insulin tolerance.

TUMOUR MARKER TESTS

PSA. CEA. CA-125. CA19-9. AFP. Lactate dehydrogenase (LDH).

TOXICOLOGY

Ethanol. Cannabis. Opiates. Benzodiazepines. Cocaine. Amphetamine.

DRUG LEVELS

Paracetamol. Salicylates. Digoxin. Lithium. Gentamicin. Carbamazepine.

MICROBIOLOGY/VIROLOGY

Bacterial. Viral. Fungal. Parasitology.

IMMUNOLOGY

Immunoglobulins. Complement levels. Autoantibody. Rheumatoid factor. Thyroid antibodies. a1AT. ACE.

MOLECULAR STUDIES

Chromosomal and DNA testing.

CROSSMATCH FOR GRUP AND SAVE PRIOR TO SURGERY AND FOR BLOOD TRANSFUSION.

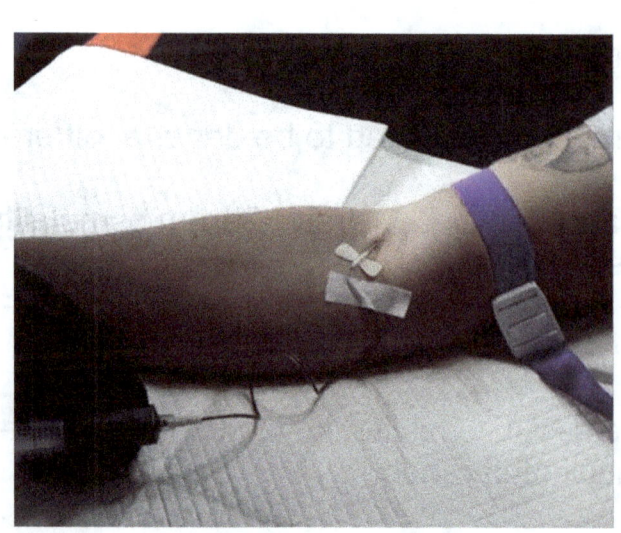

BY NICKY PEARCE

TUBES, BOTTLES AND ORDER OF DRAW

For official order of draw, you must consult the policies or your particular location for the exact policy as this may vary depending on where you are. However, there is a basic order which you must follow. Otherwise, the test results may be affected. If you are unsure, your should as the medical laboratory scientific officer, nurse or doctor.

BLOOD CULTURE BOTTLES

Always draw Aerobic first, then Anaerobic. If there is insufficient blood to fill both culture bottles, use the Aerobic bottle only.

Make sure these tests are completed before antibiotics are given otherwise there is a risk of false negative results.

Make sure drips are stopped at least 30 minutes before you take any blood, and if you have to use a cannula port to obtain a sample, make sure it is flushed with sterile saline first.

LIGHT BLUE TUBE (Sodium Citrate)
(HAEMATOLOGY FOR CLOTTING SYSTEMS)

Fill to line and invert 3-4 times. This bottle is next in line for order of draw.

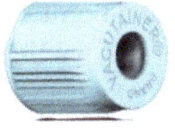

Used to test; Coagulation. D-dimer. Thrombophilia screen.

INR. International standard for Prothrombin Time PT extrinsic pathway.
Activated partial thromboplastin time (APTT). Intrinsic pathway.

RED TUBE (Silica. Which acts as a clot activator).
(BIOCHEMISTRY MAINLY. MICROBIOLOGY. SEROLOGY).
Fill to line and invert 5 - 6 times.

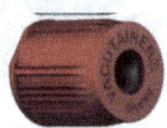

Used in sensitive tests including hormones, toxicology, drug levels, bacterial and viral serology.

LIGHT GREEN TUBE
(Lithium Heparin / Separator Gel) Fill to line and invert 8 - 10 times.

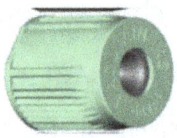

Can be used in routine Biochemistry, but most hospitals us yellow/gold tubes. Can be used for blood ethanol so long as it's not used for legal reasons.

DARK GREEN TUBE
(Lithium Heparin) Fill to line and invert 8 - 10 times.

Used for Ammonia. Insulin. Renin and Aldosterone. Aluminium. Gut hormones. Amino acids. Homocysteine. Chromosomal tests.

PURPLE TUBE
(EDTA) (HAEMATOLOGY) 1ml for FBC and full tube for ESR. Invert 8 - 10 times.

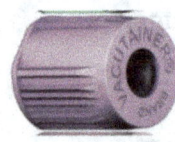

Full blood count (FBC). Erythrocyte sedimentation rate (ESR). Blood film (parasites). Reticulocytes. Red cell folate. Monospot test for EBV. HbA1C for diabetic control. Parathyroid hormone (PTH). Viral PCR. G6PD. ACTH levels. Porphyra. Fasting gut hormone screen.

BLUE TUBE
(EDTA = PLAIN) (HAEMATOLOGY) Fill to line. Invert 8 - 10 times.

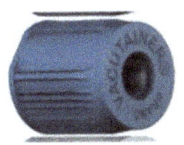

Used to check trace elements. Copper. Zinc. Selenium. Iodine. Aluminium. Long term total parenteral nutrition (TPN).

GREY TUBE
(Flouride Oxalate) (BIOCHEMISTRY) Minimum 1ml. Invert 8 - 10 times.

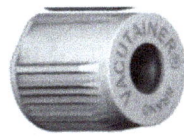

Glucose. Glucose tolerance testing. Lactate. DKA.

PINK TUBE
(SAME AS THE PURPLE BUT USED SPECIFICALLY FOR TRANSFUSION LAB). (EDTA). 1 ml minimum but more is preferred by most labs.
Invert 8 - 10 times).

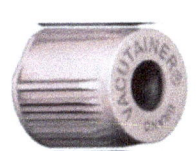

These tubes are used only for Group and Save (G&S). Used before operations where the blood group of the patient is confirmed and saved in case they require transfusion.

Crossmatch (XM). Is tested the same as above e.g. blood is typed, but is then matched to specific units of blood, platelets or other products for transfusion. THIS TUBE MUST BE LABELLED IN HANDWRITING!!!

ORDER OF DRAW

1, Culture bottles (Aerobic first, then Anaerobic).

2, Light Blue (Sodium Citrate).

3, Red (Silica Clott Activator).

4, Gold or Light Green (Lithium/Separator Gel).

5, Purple (EDTA only 1ml used for FBC).

   Navy Blue (EDTA larger tube used for other tests. Trace elements. TPN).

6, Grey (Flouride Oxalate).

7, Pink (Group and save. Cross-match etc).

PERFORMANCE CRITERIA
(ROUTINE CHECK-LIST)

1, Triage and prepare your workflow.

2, Prepare yourself to look professional. Maintaining own personal hygiene, clean ironed uniform, hair, nails, breath mints, minimal jewellery and makeup.

3, Prepare your area and equipment according to hygiene and infection control protocols. Documenting as appropriate as you go e.g. initialising cleaning rotas, sterilisation records, checking batch numbers and expiry dates.

4, Gather administrative paperwork ready, and go through it. Put in order of triage as necessary.

5, Greet the patient, introduce yourself and explain what you are there to do, also asking the patient for their consent verbally.

6, I.D. the patient in accordance with local policies and procedures e.g. check the hospital wristband or ask the patient to confirm their name and date of birth and check against your administration that you have the correct person.

7, Wash your hands, and then explain to the patient that you're going to have a feel around at the veins in their arms to pick a suitable one. Also ask the patient where they normally get their blood taken from, they may have a preference and they will know the best place to go.

8, Always ask the patient each time you do something so that you keep getting their consent. Apply the tourniquet and palpate the veins to choose one. Once you have selected one, release the tourniquet immediately so as not to cause pooling.

9, Apply a suitable cleanser to the chosen area.

10, Wash your hands or use alcohol gel before putting on gloves.

11, Get a sterile field out, ready to place any equipment on if needed. e.g. for Blood Cultures.

12, Unpack and assemble your syringes, needles, and tube in front you the patient so that they can see you are using sterile, pre-packed equipment etc. Then place the tubes in the order of draw.

13, Again re-check you have consent by asking if they are ok to proceed.

14, Apply a tourniquet, and watch for the vein that you chose to fill up.

15, Visualise where you are going to insert the needle and apply tension just below to stabilise the vein.

16, Swiftly insert the needle, bevel pointing up at an angle of approx 30-45 degrees until you see a flash of blood come up the needle window.

17, Stabilise the needle and tube. Then insert the first vacutainer. Or if using a syringe, pull back slowly.

18, Collect the amount needed according to the lab requirements, inverting the vacutainer tubes as you remove them.

19, When you insert your last tube, a few seconds later release the tourniquets so that you don't get a pooling of excess blood after you withdraw the needle from the vein. This will prevent bruising and haematomas.

20, Once complete, withdraw the needle, and apply cotton wool and pressure as you withdraw the needle. You can ask the patient to hold the cotton wool and apply pressure whilst you dispose of the needle immediately into the sharps bin.

21, Complete the forms, and label the bottles. Then place them into the appropriate tube trays or plastic envelopes etc, according to local policy for transportation.

22, Check the patient's arm, and apply some hypoallergenic tape over the cotton wool or a plaster.

23, NOTE that Group and cross-match tubes need to be handwritten.

24, Thank the patient, and make them comfortable again before disposing of any expendables.

25, Remove gloves and wash your hands again before leaving.

26, Move on to the next patient or transport the specimens back to the lab.

These are the official performance criteria to pass the Universal College of Health Sciences Phlebotomy Certificate Level 3.

You must complete a minimum of 10 witnessed, successful blood draws before undertaking this unsupervised.

Using a simulation arm is recommended to help you gain the appropriate hand-eye coordination and procedural flow before undertaking live blood draws.

For accredited online training courses in Phlebotomy, Peripheral I.V. Cannulation and more visit www.uchsc.co.uk

Join our Facebook groups; PHLEBOTOMY TRAINING UK

YouTube Channel "Nicky Pearce".

SHARPS INJURY

If a sharps injury occurs follow this procedure.

1, STOP immediately and make and squeeze the area to make it bleed into a clean tissue, cotton wool or swab.

2, Go to the sink and remove your gloves. Wash the area in clean running water whilst squeezing it.

3, Wash the area with antibacterial soap.

4, Dry area and put a clean sterile plaster/dressing on. Before putting on gloves and continuing the procedure.

5, After you have completed the procedure, report the accident in the appropriate book, form and supervisor etc.

6, You will be referred to occupational health for testing and treatments as soon as possible. If you're working in a hospital they will send you to A&E department for testing and prophylactic treatment.

Watch our Sharps Injury First Aid Video at our YouTube channel "Nicky Pearce"

APPENDIX DIAGRAMS

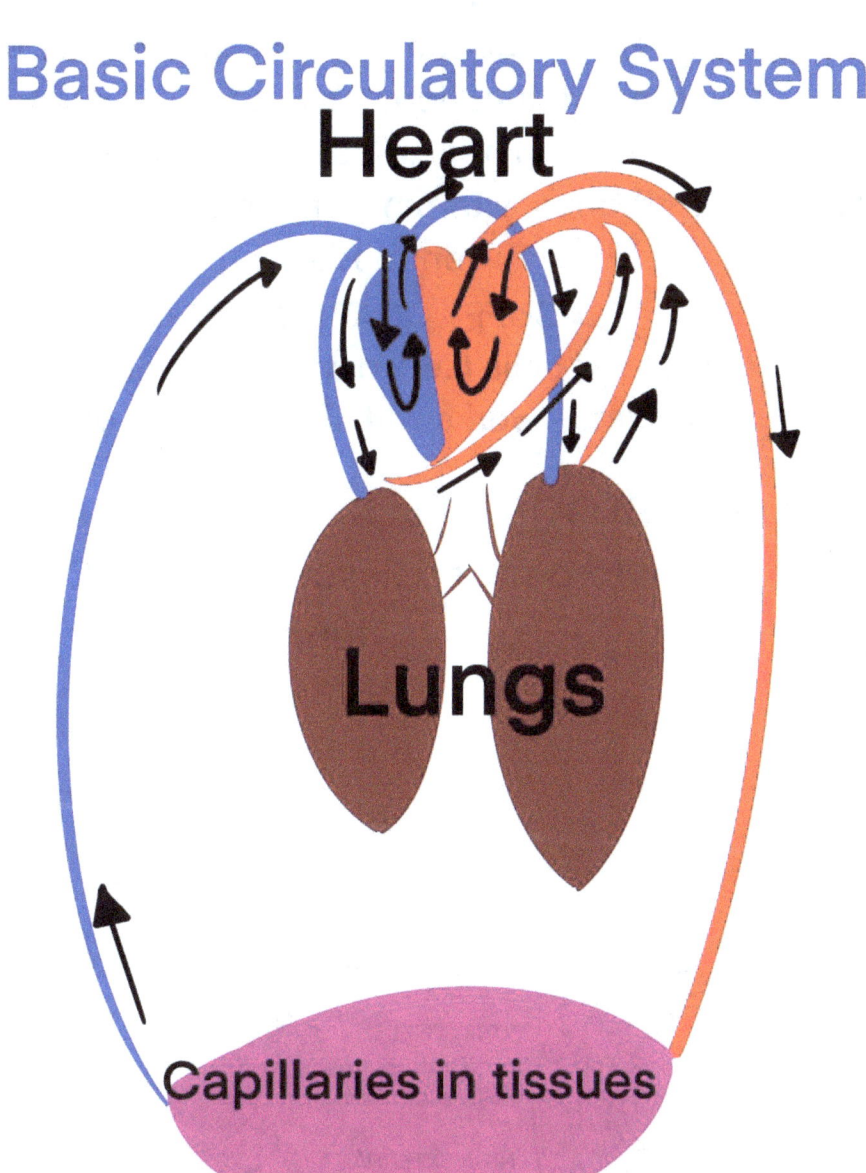

Basic Circulatory System
Heart

Lungs

Capillaries in tissues

Arteries take oxygenated blood to the tissues and organs. Veins return the blood back to the heart where it's pumped back to the lungs to be re-oxygenated and repumped back around the body again.

Normal Blood Composition

Plasma = 91% Water.

7% Proteins (Albumin 55%. = volume. Globulins 38%. immune function. Fibrinogen 7% Clotting).

1.5% electrolytes, trace elements, glucose, hormones, vitamins, amino acids, urea, antibodies.

BUFFY COAT LAYER 1%.
White blood cells (Leucocytes) = Immune defence.
Platelets - works with fibrinogen in clotting.

RED BLOOD CELLS, Erythrocytes. = Carries oxygen to perfuse tissues and CO_2 back to the lungs.

Plasma liquid

Cellular

55%

45%

Normal

Dr Nicky J Pearce.

BLOOD VESSEL STRUCTURE

Artery

Vein

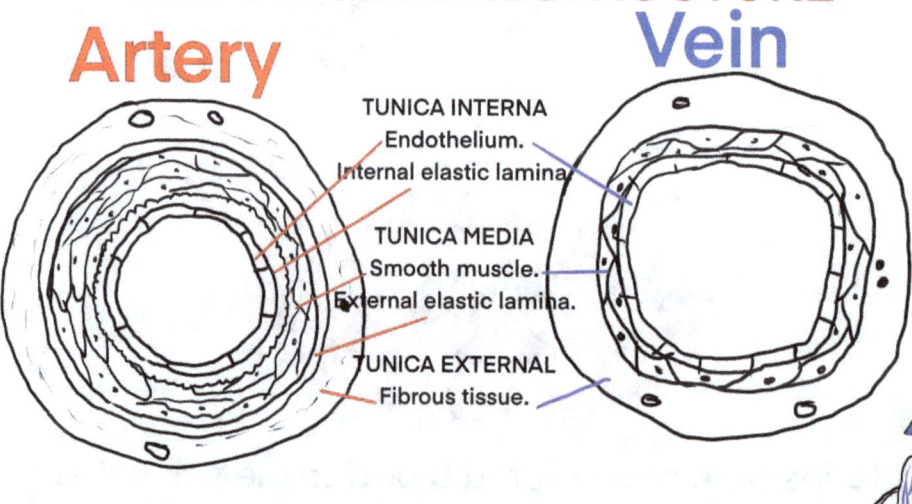

TUNICA INTERNA
Endothelium.
Internal elastic lamina.

TUNICA MEDIA
Smooth muscle.
External elastic lamina.

TUNICA EXTERNAL
Fibrous tissue.

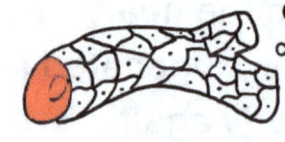

Capillaries are 1 cell thick to allow diffusion into tissues.

Red blood cell

Dr Nicky J Pearce.

Veins have valves to prevent back flow. Veins, arteries and nerves are usually found together. Some arteries are deeper.

BLOOD VESSELS

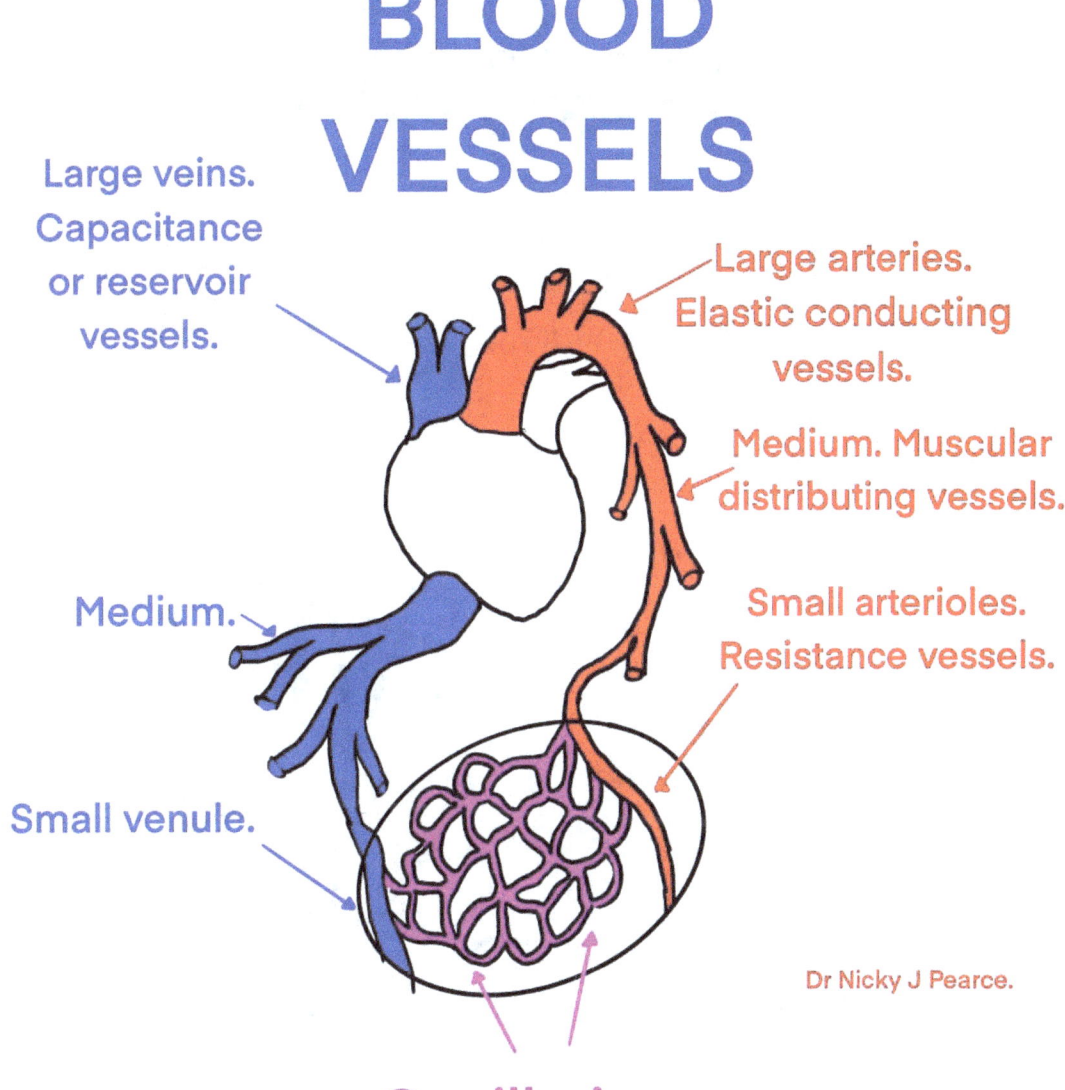

Large veins. Capacitance or reservoir vessels.

Large arteries. Elastic conducting vessels.

Medium. Muscular distributing vessels.

Medium.

Small arterioles. Resistance vessels.

Small venule.

Dr Nicky J Pearce.

Capillaries.
Larger capillaries are sinusoids.

VEIN ANATOMICAL LOCATIONS

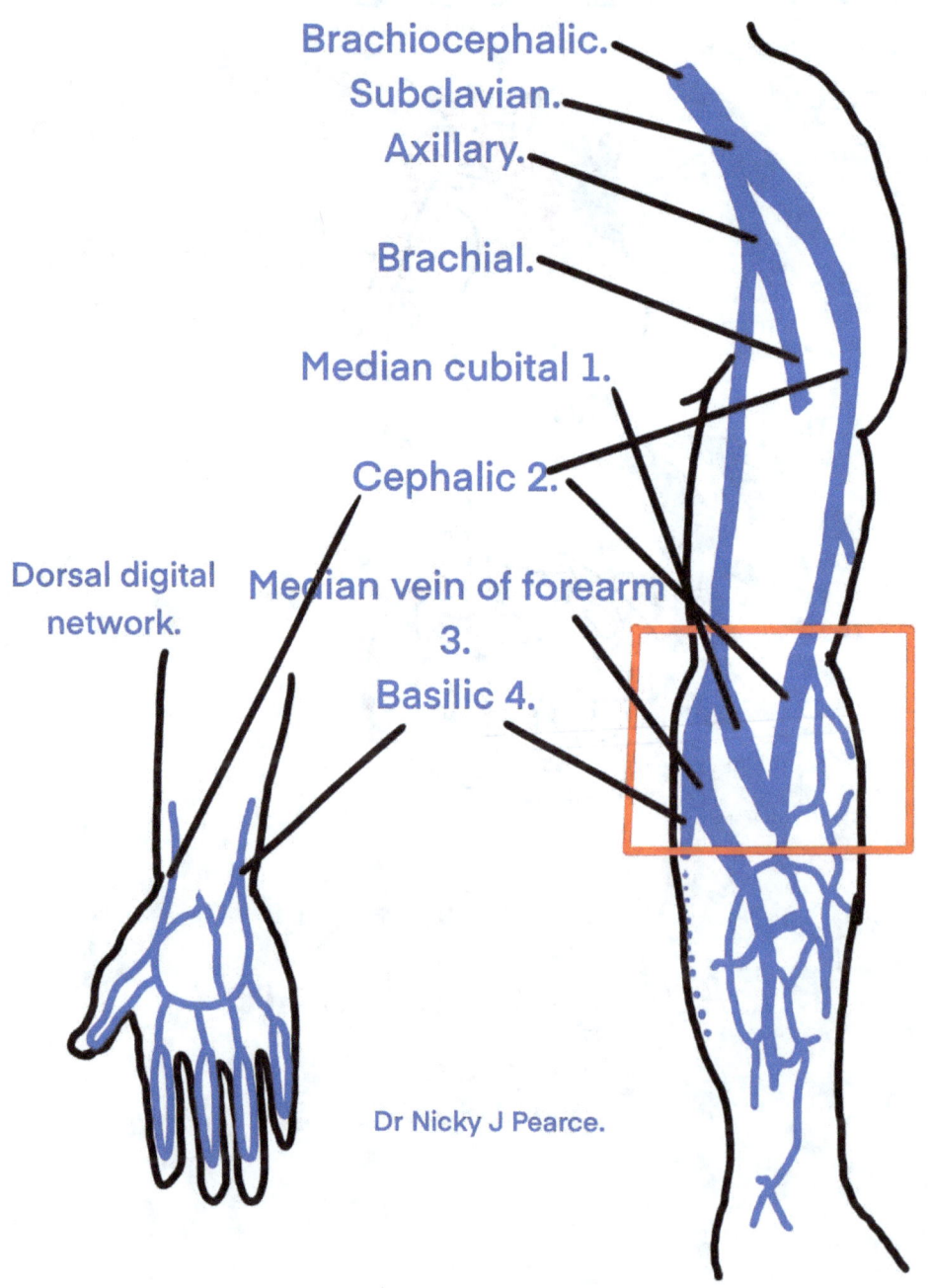

Brachiocephalic.
Subclavian.
Axillary.
Brachial.
Median cubital 1.
Cephalic 2.
Dorsal digital network.
Median vein of forearm 3.
Basilic 4.

Dr Nicky J Pearce.

Thanks to everyone who helped and supported me in making this textbook.

I hope you find it useful. If you have any suggestions we would love to hear them.

Dr, Nicky Pearce

Author and Publisher

UNIVERSAL COLLEGE OF HEALTH SCIENCES UK

GLASGOW

SCOTLAND

UNITED KINGDOM

E. uchsc_ac_uk@hotmail.co.uk

W. www.uchsc.co.uk

www.ingramcontent.com/pod-product-compliance
Lightning Source LLC
Chambersburg PA
CBHW080612220526
45466CB00010B/3325